Rocko Jay Solid

Dr. Anthony Chaffee Why we are carnivores

...and how plants try to poison you.

The science and evidence supporting our real ancestral diet.
Featuring Dr. Thomas Seyfried.

Revised Transcripts

25% of the royalties will go to Prof. Dr. Thomas Seyfrieds cancer research! See KetoForCancer.net

P.S.: Any review would be GREATLY appreciated to get the Low-Carb message out!

TABLE OF CONTENTS

Chapter 1

    Why we are carnivores   3

Chapter 2

    Carnivore for Beginners. How to start a carnivore diet   56

Chapter 3

    Plants are trying to kill you!   65

Chapter 4

    The hard facts about cancer and diet With Prof. Thomas Seyfried   86

    Other Summary Books   133

    Sources   137

Chapter 1

Why we are Carnivores

The topic of my presentation is "Why we are carnivores". This is just the arguments and evidence behind the fact that biologically humans *are* carnivores - what this means and why it matters.

First, we should really define our terms. So what is a carnivore, what is an herbivore, what is an omnivore?

A herbivore is just something that just eats only plants, pretty straightforward. A carnivore is something that that eats almost only meat. And an omnivore is something that eats both plants and meat.

But I don't think that's a very tight definition because felines are known as obligate carnivores... because almost every plant will kill them or cause serious harm. And yet, they can eat some plants. Domestic cats are fed grain and plant-based kibble which is obviously showing that they can survive on some plant food as well. So does that make them an omnivore? I don't think so.

I think what we need to define here is *what is optimal for the animal*, what is best for them to eat and survive on in the wild. We can also think of omnivore in another way. I think the really only good working functional definition of the word omnivore would be one of two things:

Either: You get as much nutrition out of both plants and animals you can eat them indiscriminately.

Or: There are things that you can only get in plants that you have to have that don't exist in meat - and there are things in meat that you have to have that don't exist in plants. And so you necessarily have to eat both.

Humans don't fall into either of those categories. We have things in meat that we have to have that we cannot get from plants, but there is nothing in plants or fungus that we have to have that we cannot get from meat.

Now, it is true that if you eat different things, you will change what your body's' requirements for different nutrients are, and this is where the RDAs come from. But these are looking at the

3

context of eating in a mixed diet - so things are very different when you're exclusively eating meat.

The evidence for this - here's just a ton of evidence we can go through these in different in different ways: Looking at things

- **Biologically**
- **Anatomically**
- **Evolutionarily**
- **Anthropologically and**
- **Metabolically**

...and the fact that plants are living things and they like to stay living things. If you eat them, they die! So all living things have a defense, while animals can run away or fight back, plants can't!

So they use poison and other mechanisms as a way to deter animals and insects from eating them. Poison being a main issue there. So why is this important?

Well, it's important because when we're talking about living optimally, you have to be able to eat the optimal nutrition. And if meat provides optimal nutrition and plants can cause harm through their defense chemicals, it is obviously not optimal to be a so-called omnivore.

Where this really plays in, is in medicine and our concept of chronic diseases - which I argue are not diseases per se: These are *toxicities* and malnutrition, really. So a toxic buildup of species-inappropriate diet and a lack of species-specific nutrition.

Namely, too many plants, not enough animal protein and fat.

You can look at this as simply as looking at animals in the zoo. Animals in the zoo, you have signs that say "Don't feed the animals!", if you feed these animals something they don't eat, they get sick.

Any proper zookeeper that knows what they're doing can tell you, if you feed an animal something that it doesn't eat in the wild that they get sick. But what do they get sick with? They get obesity, heart disease, diabetes, cancer, autoimmune diseases, arthritis and all the rest of them.

These things don't exist in the wild, and they don't exist in animals that eat their optimal, appropriately specific biologically adapted diet.

Dogs and cats are known carnivores and yet we give them grain- and plant-based kibble. Because it's cheap and it's a filler - and they get sick too and they get all these same diseases. We get all these same diseases.

In fact, veterinarians are now are saying, they're showing, that domestic animals are having a much higher rate of so-called human diseases... they're getting all the diseases that we are getting. Like diabetes, like cancer. And that this is something that has been increasing dramatically.

You can make different arguments, but it correlates perfectly with the advent of packaged dog food becoming the main way of feeding animals, and these diseases started rising precipitously. And the average life expectancy dropped precipitously.

The average life expectancy of a Golden Retriever in America in the 1970s was 17 years, now it's 9 years! Some people might say this is because of aggressive breeding programs... but the Golden Retriever was already a pure breed! I don't see how just making more of them is going to cut their life expectancy in half, without causing any major problems in other directions.

Why we are Carnivores - Biologically:

We can look at this in a number of different ways but we can start from our teeth. Our teeth have changed dramatically in the last 8 million years, becoming smaller and smaller - because we're chewing softer and softer foods. We're not chewing on sticks all day like a like a gorilla does.

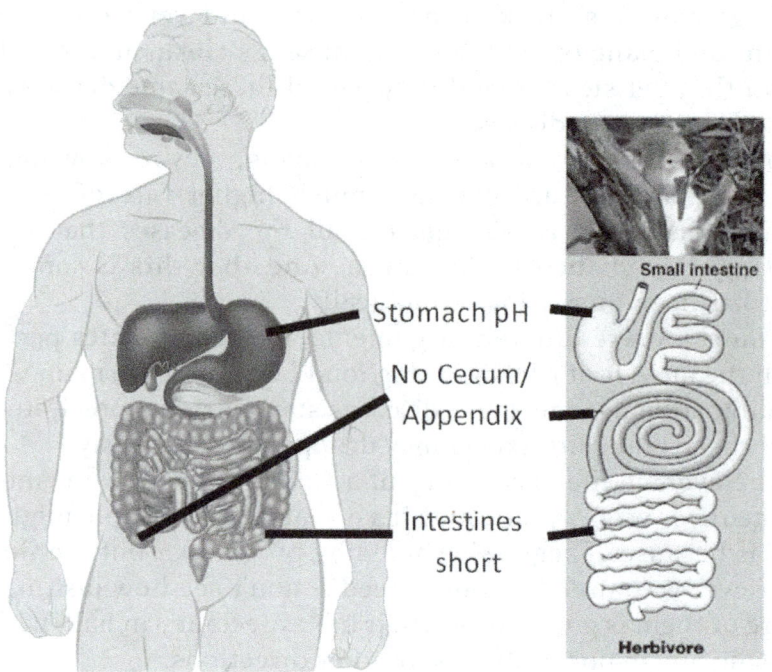

So we're getting carnivorous adaptations to our teeth and our brains. Our brains are growing bigger because we can support a bigger brain, and we also need a bigger brain to figure out how to get animal sourced protein and nutrition.

Very simple, because we cannot take down a mastodon with our bare hands, we're not going to take down an elk with our bare hands and we're not going to be able to rip it up and eat it as well. That's why we had to develop tools and tactics, and that's why our brains grew instead of our claws and our teeth. That's why we live in houses and lions don't.

That's why we developed our intelligence. And chimpanzees and gorillas didn't. But then just looking at the GI tract, you go down to our stomach: Our stomach PH is very low, it's around 1.4, 1.5. And other carnivores are around like 2, lions are usually around 2.

You look at buzzards and vultures and scavenger animals, they're around the 1.4, 1.5 range. That's because the food that they're eating has a high bacterial load, so they need to be able to kill off that bacteria to they don't get sick.

We in our evolutionary past seem to have come from a scavenger background, where we were just eating off the remains of the kills that another, more physically adapted animal had left after eating.

This is actually where the original stone tools came from, using big large pound stones to crack open the skulls of these animals and get at the brains. Because it was very nutritious, very high calorie and fat content.

But that's what we had to adapt, we had to adapt that high stomach PH, simply because we had to eat meat that had a lot of bacterial load. Even more recently, without refrigeration, people would be eating meat that was not fresh anymore.

They'd try to store and dry meat, but things would go off, things would go bad and you'd have to be able to contend with that high bacterial load.

Then, you look at the fact that we have 5 organs working in concert just to absorb fat!

So

- our stomach starts breaking down food by process of digestion
- our liver makes bile
- our gallbladder stores that bile
- our pancreas makes things like lipase and other enzymes, that break down the food and break down the fat into digestible absorbable products, and
- then that bile emulsifies the fatty acids and your small intestine absorbs it

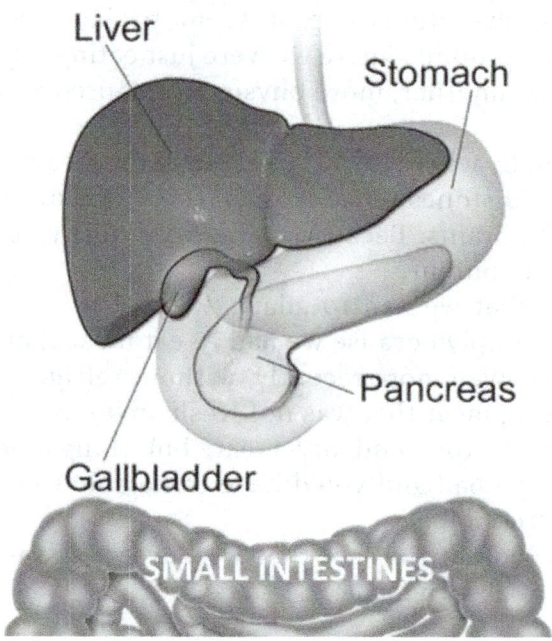

Okay, so you have 5 organs working in concert just to absorb fat. If fat weren't really, really important, our body would not do this! It wouldn't waste its time and energy. This is a very high energy demand to keep these organs functioning in that process of absorbing fat.

So if fat wasn't extremely important, we would not be spending all this energy and coordination in order to absorb it.

The other fact is that we cannot break down fiber. All herbivores that eat high fiber diets, they get actually most of their nutrition from the breakdown of that fiber. The bacteria in their guts actually feed on the fiber.

There are no vertebrate animals that can break down fiber, so they have to cultivate these bacteria which break down the fiber and actually eat the fiber - and that's what *they* get their nutrition from.

Then they expel and excrete short chain fatty acids, that's a waste product of these bacteria. And that's what the animal absorbs. And these are 100% saturated fats!

Even gorillas that just eat green leaves, they get about 70 % of their calories from saturated fat, cows get as much as 80% of their calories from saturated fat because they're much more efficient at breaking these things down.

Then those bacteria break down and die off and the animal absorbs those and gets the protein from those bacteria. So that's what they are actually eating!

We don't have that ability anymore. We've lost that millions of years ago. And this is evidenced by the fact that we have what's called an appendix. Which in other primates and other animals who are hindgut digesters is actually a very, very long cecum.

That's where fiber will actually pack down into and break down into short chain fatty acids. That's where they get the majority of their nutrition and their calories. We don't have that ability anymore.

The appendix is a vestigial cecum. Vestigial meaning that millions of years ago, it used to be this large organ that could do this... but since we haven't used it in millions upon millions of years, it has shriveled up and gone away.

Because your gut has a very high energy demand, so if you're not using part of your intestine, it is really holding you back and wasting energy... which is death in the wild.

You can also look at this as far as colon disease and diverticulosis. Diverticulosis has been shown to have only a few correlating events. So constipation ,a high fat diet and meat diets, all these sorts of things have no association with diverticulosis. In fact, there's a study showing with thousands of patients, and thousands of colonoscopies, looking at what factors were associated with this:

They found the only things that had even an association with diverticulosis - which is sort of the out pouching and breakdown of your distal colon, this can get infected and have problems, you can die from this, you have to get part of your colon removed, you have to have a colostomy bag...

The only things that were associated with diverticulosis, which could then turn to diverticulitis, was increased fiber and increased number of bowel motions a day.

So the more fiber people ate, the more people defecated, the more likely they were to have colon disease, and the breakdown and failure of their colon.

Because that's how I think about it, I think of this as organ failure, such as heart failure. Your heart is beating against a very high pressure gradient for years and decades on end, and eventually it just goes "That's it, I give up" and it starts to break apart and break down. That's heart failure.

Well, I look at diverticulosis as colon failure: You have overworked this organ and it's just run out of life. it's just run out of miles, and it's just going to start falling apart now and not work as well as it would have otherwise.

Even when people do get diverticulitis or appendicitis or cancer, anastomoses and other sorts of bowel issues, you will see general surgeons and colorectal surgeons putting people on what is called a low residue diet. That's just a low fiber diet and that's because they want to rest the bowel.

So they don't want the bowel working and expending all this effort and energy and pushing and squeezing and peristalting to get rid of this stuff, right? Because they want the bowel to just heal and rest. You don't want to overwork it.

Okay, but everyone's saying that fiber is good for you, that that peristalsis and moving and motion, all that stuff is really good for the bowel and this is beneficial for you. If that's true, then why do we whenever there's a problem rest the bowel and avoid fiber? And that helps the bowel.

If fiber is going to help the bowel and it's good for the bowel, then it should be good in those circumstances as well! That never really made sense to me because you're causing harm in a harmed state, why is that not causing a harm or overworking and overusing that organ in a non-pathological state? That never really made sense to me.

These people will say "Don't eat fiber!" - but then when this is done "Oh, you better eat fiber, because that's what's going to protect you!" That makes absolutely no sense! And the only reason people are saying this is just because they've been trained to say this their entire life, and they haven't actually thought about it.

Also think about this, this is waste material. This is going out.

It's being excreted, that means your body can't use it. That means your body didn't want it and it wants to get it out. If fiber was so good for us, why is our body just pushing it out at all costs?

It actually isn't good for us, it actually causes harm to us. It causes micro-abrasions in the gut lining, causes increased mucus secretion and inflammatory responses as well.

It also blocks the absorption of nutrients in our small intestine and makes it impossible for our body to absorb everything that we're eating. How is that beneficial?

How is that evolutionarily selective? Why is it that if you're eating something and you're blocking your body from absorbing the nutrients, that this provides an advantage somehow? That doesn't make any sense either.

So you have to think about these things on first principles. And when you start looking that like that in this direction, these things start becoming a little more obvious.

Then you have IBDs, irritable bowel diseases such as Crohn's and ulcerative colitis. There are studies, actually going back to the 1890s, showing that if you put people on a pure red meat and water diet, that you actually reverse these and stop these processes from happening.

Dr. JH Salisbury - of the Salisbury steak - has actually shown this, he wrote a whole book about it! Even as recently as 1975 Dr. Volklin, who's a gastroenterologist, also reiterated this and wrote a book called *The Stone Age Diet*. Arguing that humans, yes, are carnivores. And if you eat as a carnivore, you will stop having gastrointestinal diseases such as Crohn's and ulcerative colitis.

More recently... because this has all been papered over, because everyone said that fat and cholesterol were bad... and so 100 years of medical literature and knowledge just gets thrown out the window and were just completely ignored after that.

But even more recently, there have been studies looking at elemental diets with IBD, Crohn's and ulcerative colitis... An elemental diet, meaning that they just take the specific macro / micro nutrients that you need, without any of the extra stuff that that comes along with this.

They found that this was better for getting people out of an acute flare-up of Crohn's and ulcerative colitis than steroids were, like Prednisolone or Prednisone.

They also looked at fasting mimicking diets. A fasting mimicking diet is just a ketogenic diet, so you're just eliminating carbohydrates, getting your metabolism into the so-called fasting state.

Which, as anyone who's listened to me before, knows that I completely disagree with: I think that is our primary metabolic state! This would be another piece of evidence to suggest that.

Because on a fasting mimicking diet, versus a carbohydrate with fiber diet, they found that people with Crohn's and ulcerative colitis stayed in remission on average 51 weeks - whereas on the carbohydrate and fiber diet they stayed in remission on average zero weeks! All right? That's not a lot of weeks!

This is already in the literature now, so you don't even need all the stuff going back 100 years, 120 years, 150 years. But it is there.

Anatomically:

Again, we spoke about teeth and how this is changing over millions and millions of years. People say that we have flat teeth because they just look flat in the front. They're not actually, they're bicuspid teeth.

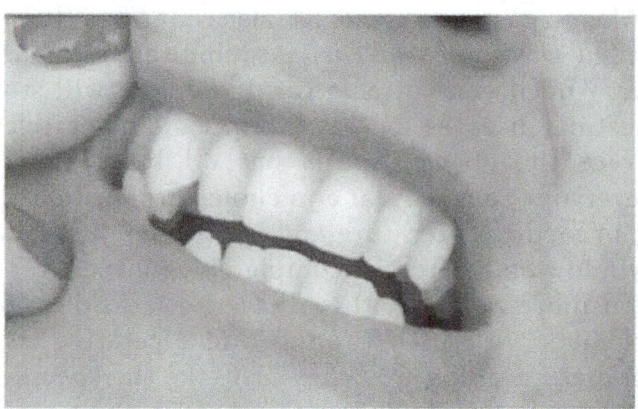

Flat teeth are like a millstone, they can slide against each other. They can grind down fibrous plants into more easily digestible mush and then you can swallow that and your body can break it down a little better.

But we actually have bicuspid teeth. So if you bite down and clench your teeth and try to move your jaw side to side it doesn't move at all. That's because we don't have flat teeth. If we had flat teeth, we would be able to make that sliding mechanism and that's what other animals with flat teeth are able to do, like horses and cows.

And again: We have smaller teeth, smaller jaws, smaller muscles of mastication. If you look at the picture of the Gorilla here:

Most of that head is actually big temporalis muscles, big muscles of mastication. The skull of a Gorilla has a huge crest going back and that's where all the muscles attach. So that's a just a ball of muscle on its head right there.

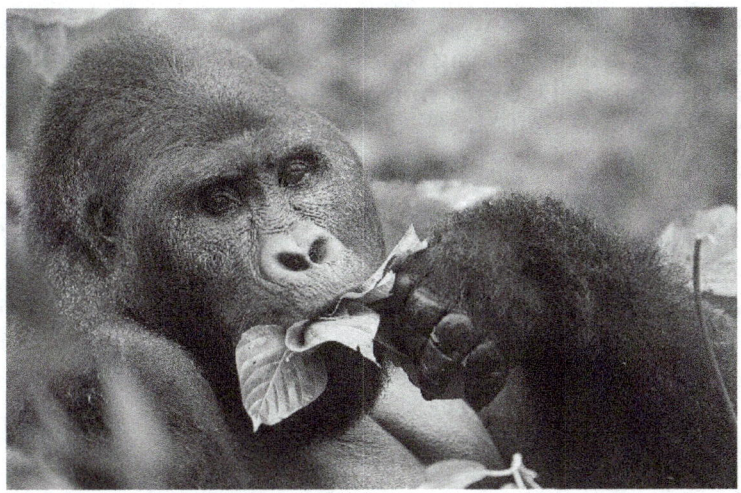

You look at our shoulders: Our shoulders have a rotational capacity that allows us to throw things very hard and very fast. Like rocks, like spears, like other weapons or boomerangs. To hunt animals, take them out and take them as food.

Chimpanzees can't do that. Chimpanzee... or Bonobo, is our closest relative really in the animal kingdom, and they don't have that capacity in their shoulders.

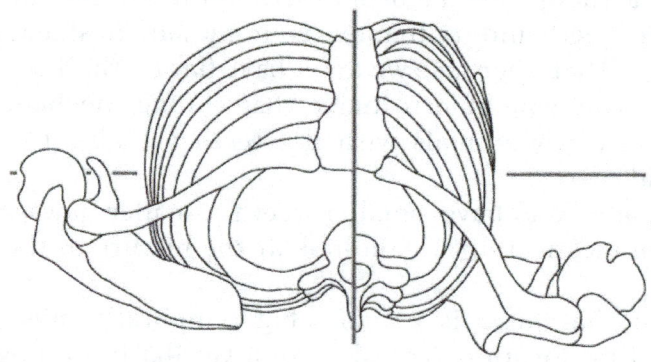

While the average adult male can throw a baseball about 60 miles an hour - and obviously people that are trained up can do much faster than that - even the strongest, most adept chimpanzees are only going to be able to throw a baseball about 20 miles an hour. That's because they don't have that rotational capacity in their shoulders.

We also have very different eyes to prey animals. This is something that we see very often in predator animals: They have these forward-facing eyes that give 3D vision, and you can focus in on your prey and you can hunt them down.

And then generally, prey animals, they have wider set eyes so that they can see in a much wider range, so they can see animals creeping up on them.

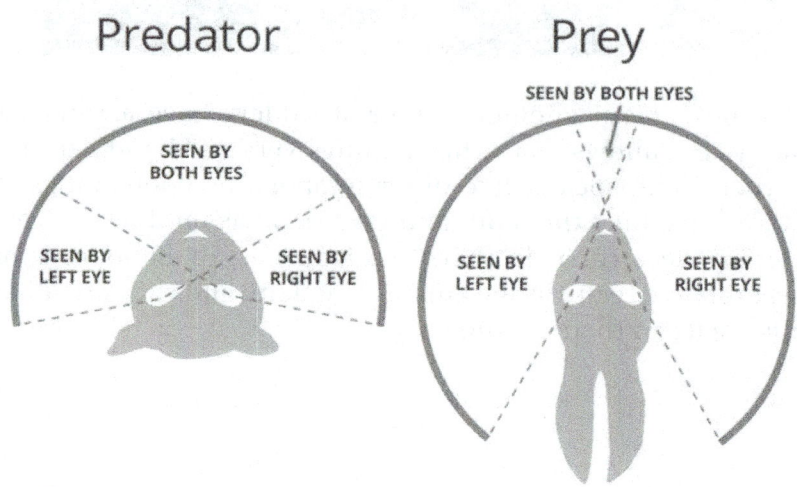

People do talk about color vision, they say "Well, color vision is to look at different colored fruits and see the differences in plants." That's possible, but it doesn't really matter because we do come from a herbivorous past, we do know that.

We don't lose a genetic trait unless there's an evolutionary advantage to do so. Unless there is an advantage to lose that color vision, then there's no point in getting rid of it.

That's why we can still move our jaws from side to side, that comes from that herbivorous past. But again, there wasn't any real advantage from not being able to move your jaw from side to side. So it ended up sticking around.

But there actually are some people that have developed color blindness. Even just red green color blindness. Why is that an advantage? Well, it's an advantage because you can see better in low light and you can actually see animals... the contrast between animals and plants a lot better. So it's actually really good for hunting.

So this has provided an adaptive advantage for hunting. But at the same time, color vision is good for other things and so it could be that it just didn't completely overshadow the ongoing benefits of color vision as well.

Evolutionarily:

As I mentioned, about 8 million years ago we broke off from other primates because we started eating meat, started eating more meat and more meat. We started having these genetic and physical adaptations, these phenotypical adaptations that we see in the fossil record.

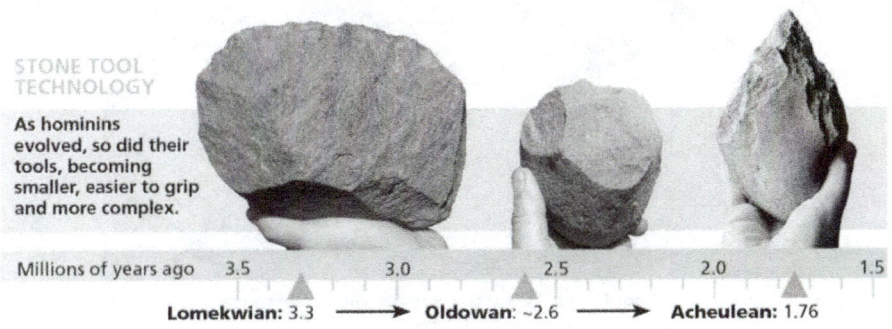

STONE TOOL TECHNOLOGY

As hominins evolved, so did their tools, becoming smaller, easier to grip and more complex.

Millions of years ago 3.5 3.0 2.5 2.0 1.5

Lomekwian: 3.3 → Oldowan: ~2.6 → Acheulean: 1.76

We started becoming more upright, we started becoming taller. We started having smaller and smaller teeth, smaller jaws, bigger brains. And we started using tools, because we had to figure out how to take down animals that outclassed us by every physical metric. Like a mastodon, or even a deer.

There aren't many people that can wrestle down a deer and beat it to death with their hands. Maybe they exist, but these things are very big, strong, powerful animals with antlers.

So we had to figure something out. We had to figure out how to take them down - and that's where tools and tactics come in.

Poundstones go back millions and millions of years. The first worked stone tool came in at around 3.3 million years ago. Those developed and became more sophisticated as the eons went by. And these were used to kill and dismember animals... and they got more and more sophisticated.

That's something that Dr. Bill Schindler speaks about in his talks and in his book *Eat like a human*. He had a great talk at Ketocon as well. It's a shame that that wasn't recorded, but you can you can find his material on Youtube as well.

What happened, that really drove us into that final stage of pure carnivorism was the ice age. Or the initiation of the ice ages, around 2, 2.5 million years ago or so. Before that, there really wasn't these ice caps, these polar ice caps. Those didn't exist further back, about 2, 2.5 million years ago.

Then we came into an ice age, which we still actually are a part of. Then these ice sheets came down, they killed off the plants, they killed off the animals that ate the plants and weren't able to survive during the ice times.

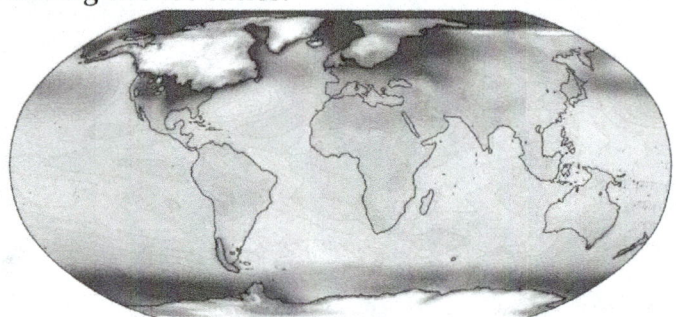

Last Glacial Maximum Surface Air Temperature
Difference from Preindustrial (°C)

-14 -12 -10 -8 -6 -4 -2 0

And really only these big megafauna, big fuzzy, furry mammals like mastodons, giant sloths and things like that, were able to survive during this period. And then the carnivores and predators that were preying on them.

Our ancestors being among them, or at least adapted enough to survive during that time, because we were eating meat and because we were eating these animals... and we became basically reliant on pure animal nutrition. Because the plants weren't available.

So our ancestors that went down that line and just went whole hog on the whole meat trade, those are the ones that survived. And those are the ones that turned into modern day humans because of that evolutionary drive and necessity for animal sourced nutrition.

We can also look at this from the fossil record and something called the stable isotope study. In stable nitrogen studies, you can find this in the bone of any animal, there you can see what that animal ate.

Basically, it builds up throughout the food chain. So animals that just eat plants, they will get a certain amount of this stable nitrogen. And then animals that eat that animal, they'll have a concentration of that nitrogen and so on. So as you go up the food chain, you get up to the top...

Like a fish that eats algae, there's a fish that eats that fish... the fish that eats that fish and so on up the chain, until you get to sharks and orca whales and things like that.

So, you can see that these are top of the food chain apex predators. And we actually see that our ancestors in early humans and even early homo sapiens and neanderthals were apex predators:

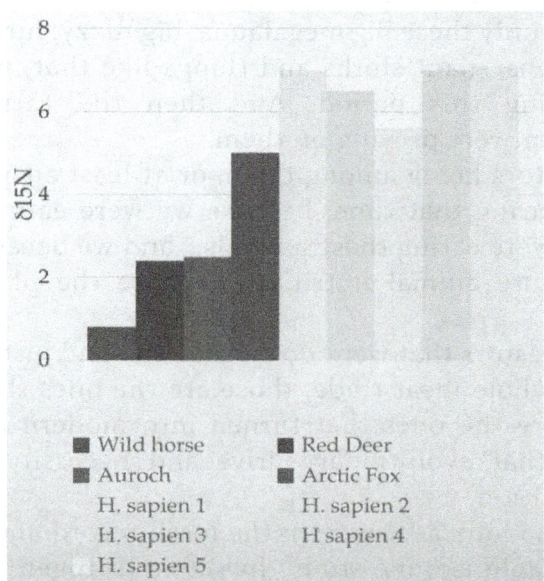

They had a higher carnivore rating than even lions, foxes, hyenas around at the same time in the same location. Okay? This is because our ancestors were eating the lions and hyenas and foxes and wolves as well!

We have looked at the stable isotope analysis of the Ancient Egyptians. Not everyone knows this, but it's thought that there are more mummies in Egypt than there are people currently alive in Egypt! This is because these were just the burial practices of Ancient Egypt.

It wasn't just the Pharaohs and the wealthy that were mummified. Certainly, the only ones buried with a fortune in gold and trinkets, but everyone was buried this way.

They looked at the stable isotope study and they found that during the agricultural revolution, post-agricultural revolution, that they were actually heavily eating grains and this actually affected their health.

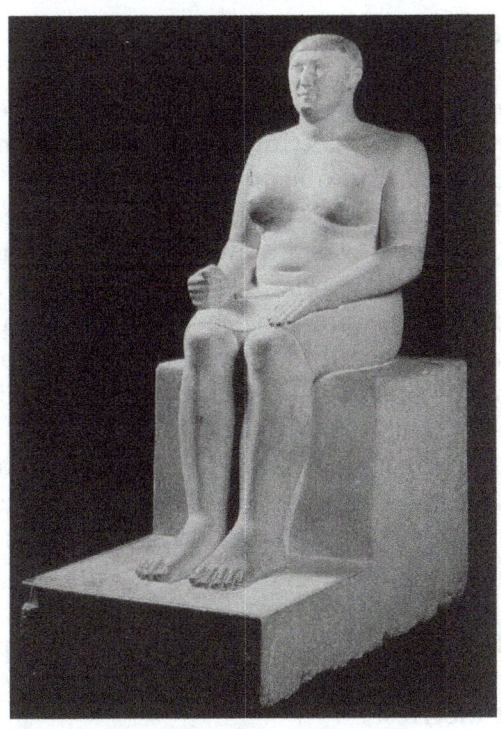

  We can look at these and we actually see atherosclerotic plaques in their hearts. This was first thought to be that the Pharaohs and wealthy were the ones eating all the rich food and they could afford meat and fat, and so obviously they were getting fatty arteries because they were eating fatty meat.
  But that actually isn't the case. When you look at the stable isotope studies, we find that the normal peasant class were eating the same amount, the same kind of food as the upper class. Just probably maybe not as much access to food... so if there was a famine or something like that, they're the ones that are going to starve first. However, they were still eating the same thing.
  And you can even see from their statuary, this is not actually the peak of human health here. This is the statue of a man who has clear gynecomastia and a pot belly Okay? So that already is showing this dysregulation of health, hormonal health in the population, just eating grains.
  So they had the original grains that they had treated and fermented or sprouted or done different things than they do

now, to get a less harmful product - and it was still causing all of these problems.

So even then, without processed sugar and refined sweets and junk food, they were still getting sick and they were still getting unwell, gynecomastia and obesity as well.

Evolutionarily, again: We look at different studies that are just all over the map. There was a major study that was done out of the University of Tel Aviv in Israel from Professor Miki Ben-Dor.

This showed that humans have been hyper carnivorous, apex predators for at least 2 million years! So again, apex predators, top of the food chain - this is what that stable isotope study shows that we actually were top of the food chain.

Apex predators don't graze! I've never seen a great white shark eat kelp for roughage. I've never seen a lion eat grass for the same reasons. This is not what apex predators do, this is not what top of the food chain animals do. They eat animals, they eat the animals below them on the food chain.

This is what the Israeli study showed as well, from Miki Ben Dor: Not only with the stable isotope study, but by many, many, many different metrics.

We showed that humans have been carnivores, apex predators, hunters. Not hunter-gatherers, hunters for at least 3 million years... and that coincides with the advent of these ice ages.

People say that "Well, when the ice ages came down, people were still eating plants they still had to do this" and you point out that like "Well, during the ice ages, there really weren't any fruits or vegetables available to people. Because it's ice!"

And they argue "Well, no. People just moved towards the equator when that happened."

That's actually completely false, that is nowhere argued in any of the scientific literature. And in fact, it's very clear from the fossil record that as the ice shelves were moving down, people were moving up! Probably because this is where their preferred prey was, which is like the mastodons and megafauna.

We can also look at the fossil record and look at what happened after the agricultural revolution. A paleo-anthropologist can actually look at a fossil, a skull and teeth, and actually tell you if a human skull was before or after the agricultural revolution.

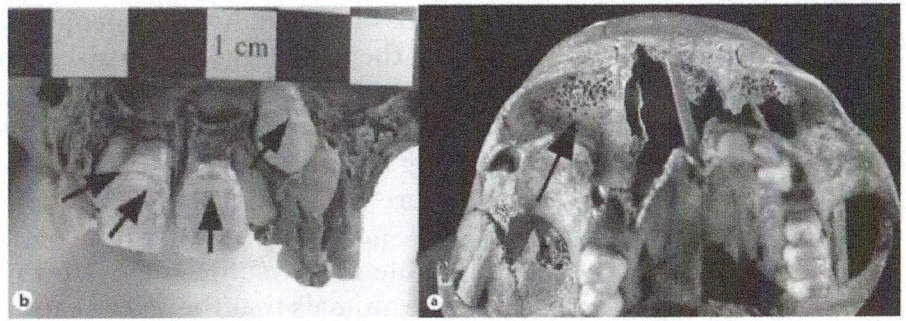

Teeth and jaws will only develop properly with proper nutrition. And so crooked teeth, small jaws, micronathia... those are all a product of malnutrition. So not getting enough of the appropriate nutrients that we need will make it impossible for our bodies to develop properly.

There are other things as well. Mouth breathing, sucking your thumb, using bottles and all that sort of stuff, they can actually change how your mouth develops. Chewing on actual food, this stimulates the development of your jaw as well.

But looking at this, just from a nutritional standpoint: You do need specific nutrients like vitamin K_1, K_2, calcium, vitamin D and so on, in order to make straight teeth.

This is published widely in dentistry journals today, that this is a phenomenon, that this is not a genetic issue. Crooked teeth are not a genetic problem. They are a nutritional problem, this is from not getting the proper nutrients.

So when we look at the fossil record before the agricultural revolution, we actually see very wide jaws with straight teeth, all of their wisdom teeth are in and comfortably so. Their jaws are big and straight and wide and pronounced. They're not these short truncated crowded jaws with crowded teeth.

Why is it that now, almost no one gets their wisdom teeth in, whereas a couple hundred years ago most people did. If they were getting proper nutrition.

People say "Well, we're revolving away from that." I am sorry, but it takes way longer to evolve than just a couple hundred years or even a couple generations. Because just a generation or two ago, not getting your wisdom teeth in was actually less common than it is now. Far less common than it is now.

When we look at height in the fossil record: Actually people in the prehistoric era were taller and they had larger brain sizes. So the average brain size of homo sapiens was 11% larger before the agricultural revolution than it is now! The Neanderthal brains are actually larger than that, going back like 50,000 years.

This is likely because even before the agricultural revolution, maybe people did start adding the -gathering part of the hunter-gatherers because they weren't able to get sufficient nutrition, sufficient fat and calories from the animals that they were eating - because the megafauna was going extinct and we had to look at other sources of nutrition to help mitigate this.

Before that, our brains were actually bigger and people were actually taller. There are areas where people were known to have been hunting mammoths and we can date these and say "Okay, these guys were mammoth hunters" and we can see this by other metrics as well, to show that that's what they were eating.

They found that that some of these populations were on average 6 foot 2 or even 6 foot 4 - and that's on average! The average height of an adult male in America is 5 foot 8 and in China, Mongolia and elsewhere, it's like 5 foot 6, 5 foot 4. That's very, very short. And that's the average, so half the population would be below that.

Not so in the areas that had an abundance of meat to eat, like these big mastodon hunters. On average about 6 foot 2 or more. So a lot of these people were much taller than that as well. The different tribes in Africa where they just eat meat, on average these guys are 6 foot 2, 6 foot 4.

The average height of a population denotes the average health of a population. And while you may have geographical differences in population... Like you have the pygmies in Africa, those guys are not that tall.

However, you do have different populations like in Asia, we have people that went through the forced famines of Mao Zedong and the other communist famines... obviously, they had stunted growth.

Then you have all these elderly Chinese people who are very short. But: Then they come over to America and they have kids who are 6 foot 4! Because this is a nutritional issue, this is not just a genetic issue.

We look at brain size as well. This is a chart of our brains growing, going back 10 million years and it's slowly creeping up.

And then you see at around 2, 2.5 million years, all of a sudden this spike up. That's because during that slow rise, we're eating more meat and more fat... and we're growing our brain because we're figuring out how to get better quality food, we're starting to figure out tools...

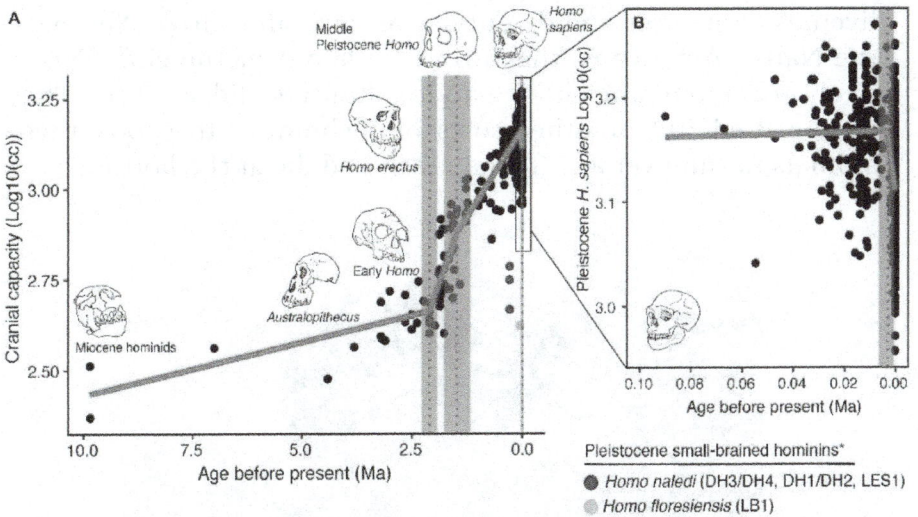

And all of a sudden, when we're basically forced to go full carnivore because we don't have any other options with the ice ages, our brain development skyrockets! And it has this exponential growth, right up until the end there.

Where you can see: Right there at the end, it all of a sudden has a sharp decline downwards. You cannot argue that that is a genetic change, that is something that happened in the environment. Genetic changes don't happen that fast.

So it's nearly a straight line when you look at it. In proportion at that small area... and then almost direct line downwards, okay? That is a sharp, sharp decline!

Something happened there, something happened that was not good for us. And if you actually look at that, that coincides with the advent of agriculture and plant-based nutrition becoming more prevalent.

Not even as dominant as it is now, just more prevalent. Okay? Before that, we were carnivores, we're living as carnivores. Then we add in plants on a wide scale – bam! Our brain size goes down! That's not good. That is a very clear piece of evidence that this is not the way we should be eating.

Anthropologically:

Looking at different populations around the world that have lived as carnivores and do survive as such and thrive: You have the Native Americans, they drove buffalo over the cliff. This is likely what our ancient mastodon hunters did as well. They maybe used fire or other sorts of techniques to spook these animals to run over a cliff, and crash and die at the bottom.

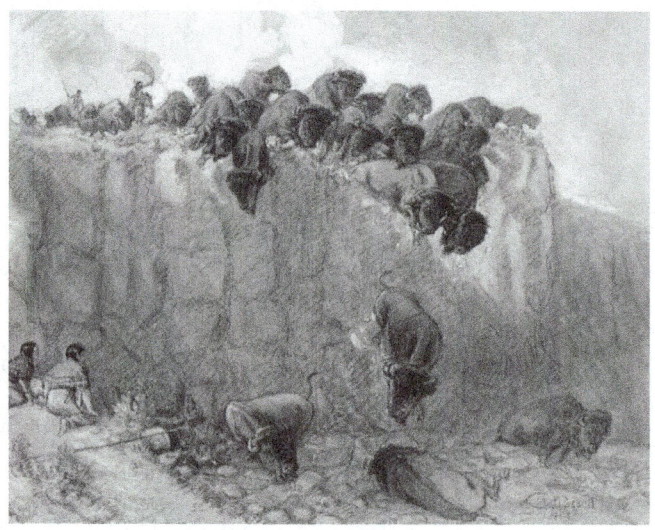

And they would use stone tools to cut them up, dry them and make pemmican in order to preserve that meat, fat and nutrition throughout the rest of the year.

They would do that, they would have one big buffalo drop a year sometimes, and they would feed their entire family and community for an entire year.

They were also very strong, very powerful, very physically and mentally dominant people. Just because they didn't have technology, they didn't have the iPhone, does not mean that they weren't intelligent. It doesn't mean that they weren't more intelligent than we are now, and they likely were.

When you have harder environments and situations to live in, it actually necessitates more intelligence and ingenuity. Now we have it pretty soft, we don't have to use our brain as much, we don't have to figure out how to survive. They did.

They actually were quite a lot taller than they are now. Dr. Stephen Phinney has talked about this multiple times. There was one example that he gave, these paintings of these Native Americans, these people were very tall and slender with large heads. And they said that these guys were actually... and this was from early 1800s, they would say that these guys were actually like 6 foot 7, 6 foot 8.

And they're like "That's not possible! Look how big their heads are, they would have been like a beach ball!" No, in fact they were and there's a lot of documentation to show that.

They actually came and met the Great White Father Thomas Jefferson who was president at the time. And Thomas Jefferson who was like 6 foot 2, he commented like "These guys were giants! They were massive with big old heads!" And big old head means big old brain. That was a commonly recorded thing.

We even have documentation of sailors coming over to the new world - and they said the natives were very brave. Talk about Indian braves, they were very brave. They had no fear.

They would just jump out into the ocean, swim out to the boat, climb up there and walk around, just look around expecting people... but naked! Didn't have anything with them.

And the captain actually wrote in his journal or whatever, that subsequently became published, that these guys

> *without a stitch of clothing on them were physical specimens. And they were more beautiful just in their nakedness than any English gentleman in their finest regalia.*

They said these people were just beautiful and beautifully built. And very tall, very strong and very muscular. This is something that we see as a rule around the world in these carnivore populations of humans.

Genghis Khan: This was an entire nation, a massive one... an entire empire that just ate carnivore! They ate horse meat, they drank horse blood, they would have some fermented milk products as well - and they dominated most of Asia and most of Europe.

This was the largest continuous empire that has ever existed - and they ran solely on a carnivorous diet. And that gave them extreme benefits and advantages to warfare and governing huge tracts of land.

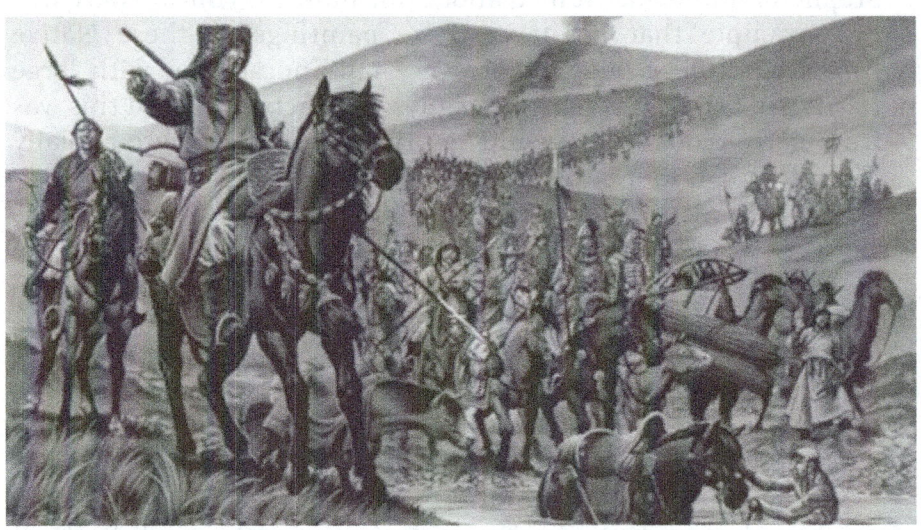

First and foremost, because they didn't need to eat 4 times a day. They didn't have to stop and cook and eat and have low energy all the time. They could go 5 days without eating, then they would eat 10 pounds of horse meat in a go and they'd be good for another 5 days. That actually routinely happened!

Or they were on a ride and they're just going and their horse would be bled, they would get some blood from the horse - and that would last them for the day or two. heir horse would make more blood, and they would just keep going. So this was a renewable resource as well, the blood of the horses. As well as the milk.

And people talk about how agriculture was just the finest advent, because this allowed us to have cities.

Well, I'm sorry: We have the largest continuous empire ever that existed on a carnivore diet. Did not need agriculture, did not need farmland, did not need to grow crops and grains - and they had the largest continuous empire that's ever existed!

The only thing that eclipsed it - as far as land mass is concerned - was the British Empire, more recently. But that was a naval power, that was scattered all over the world. This was one huge chunk of the world. What is now Russia is really some of the remnants of the Mongol Empire.

Look at a map sometime and google that and see, just how big this empire was. And then see for yourself if you believe the whole idea, that you had to have grains and agriculture to have a civilization or cities.

The Native Americans did the same thing: There was a city that was found abandoned... because 95% of the Native Americans died off through diseases brought over from Europe accidentally, in the early 1600s.

They found this city in what is now St. Louis, that had buildings and structures that were estimated to be able to house one million full-time residents. And they had trade routes going off in 5 major directions, all across the continent, in order to bring in food, trade, goods and so forth. Right there, there was a city, a million people in it... that's the population size of ancient Rome. So it can be done.

Then you have the Inuits, Eskimos. These and other populations that live up in the arctic circle: There's no plants to access, even if they wanted to... which they actually don't. There was a chronicle, a journal of a New England settler and explorer that spoke about this, where... a couple months out of the year, in the more southern reaches of Canada...

"The western people said that 'Okay, I understand that during the winters, they're very harsh, there are no plants, you can't cultivate anything. So you have to just eat meat! But in the two, three months of the fall, surely they can live off the bounty of the land!'" Which is how he phrased it.

And he said "But they didn't! They did not do that! What they did was they ate meat, even in those times that they could have grown crops."

Now people say "Well, they would have ate berries" and this, that and the other..."

Especially when you go up further north, there really weren't berries accessible. And the ones that were, these little lingonberries, those are extremely sour. And in fact most of them didn't like them, they didn't want to eat them.

So, the gathering part of that hunter-gatherer motif was at most 2 months out of the year... for things that no one really ate. Like lingonberries.

You have the Masai in Africa and many other populations and tribes out there as well: They still just eat meat.

Look at these guys: They're tall, they're slender, they're strong. There were studies back in the 1980s looking at the Masai, saying like "These guys are just built like olympic athletes. They can run forever, they never get tired, they never run out of energy. They just go go go."

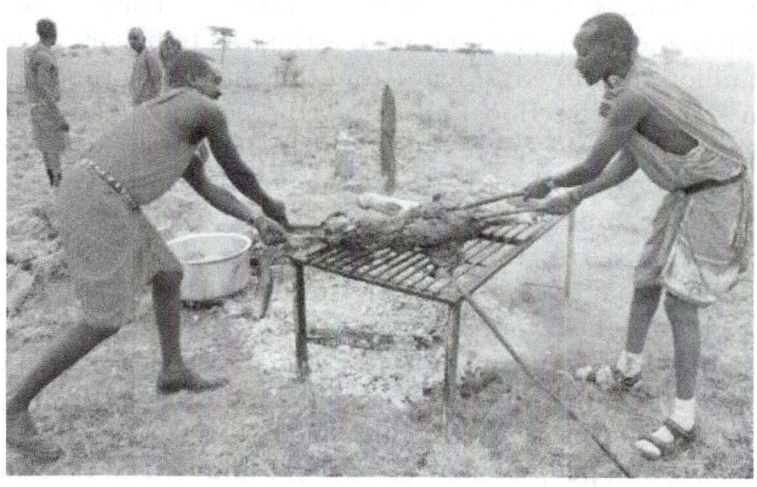

They thought that this must be because of the amount of exercise they did, because this was right when people were saying that fat, cholesterol, killed you - made you fat and sick.

Yet, these guys were eating a lot of fat, they were drinking blood, drinking fatty milk. Which... the milk of their livestock is about 8 % milkfat, as ours is about 3.5 to 4.5% from cow's milk.

These guys were extremely healthy and extremely fit. So they said "Well, it must be because of their exercise level. They're just out there, they're out there being fit. " And so they did a study and looked:

They found that "Well, actually: No! Not really." On average, their daily exercise and energy expenditure through athletic endeavors was 1.6 times that of the average American. Which was always said to be very sedentary, very slothful, a bunch of couch potatoes with belly fat and no cardiovascular health. That sort of throws that theory out the window as well.

The Native Australian Aborigines: There's so much documentation about how these guys were hunters, exclusively. They knew which plants that they could eat, if they had to. But they didn't, unless they had to, or to use medicinally. They were hunters, they hunted kangaroo and other animals, and they exclusively ate meat.

And they were very healthy. They're very tall, they're actually, they have very tall slender builds. Just like the Masai, very muscular and trim. And now, that is not the case anymore.

Remember, I was talking about these human diseases. Those were really called *the diseases of the West* previously. So previously, diseases of the West were things like obesity, diabetes, heart disease, all these sorts of things. Heart disease really wasn't described until the 1900s...

But people getting these sorts of diseases and getting sick, they only saw these in western populations.

And I remember learning as a kid that when eating a western diet, Native Americans were 4 times as likely to get all the Western diseases, chronic diseases, that we get today. Like heart disease, diabetes, cancer, obesity as well.

And I remember thinking at the time "Well, doesn't that mean that the food is causing the disease? Because if they don't eat the food, they don't get the disease - and we eat the food and we get the disease, we just get it a lower rate!"

"What is a western diet versus a non-western diet? What are they eating that we're not and vice versa?" They didn't say it at the time, but you later learned, that they were eating just a pure carnivore diet. Maybe some plants, sometimes, if they had to. Maybe. But generally, they didn't!

The vast majority of what they ate was just meat. The Australian Aborigines were no different.

In fact, when I first came to Australia to practice medicine, I learned right away that, basically, the health of the Australian

Aborigines was quite poor. I was told that whenever treating an aboriginal patient that whatever their age said on their chart, just to add 20 years to that. Because that is just how quickly they age.

So if you had someone who's 45, you basically consider the diseases that someone would get in a 65 year old, because that is just what you generally see. And so if you're seeing like a range of diseases or cancers from 60 to 70, or 60 to 80 years, you can actually look at that from 40 to 60 in the aboriginal population.

That is seriously affecting them. That is because they didn't have exposure to the agricultural revolution like European populations did, and others around Asia and India as well, and northern Africa in certain parts. These people are going to be much more affected by the plant toxins that exist to defend these plants against predation.

They are going to become more hurt. This again, goes back to the fact that these are not diseases! This is a poison-dose relationship! When you remove this substance, these diseases go away. That is a toxin / toxic relationship, that is not a disease relationship. Okay?

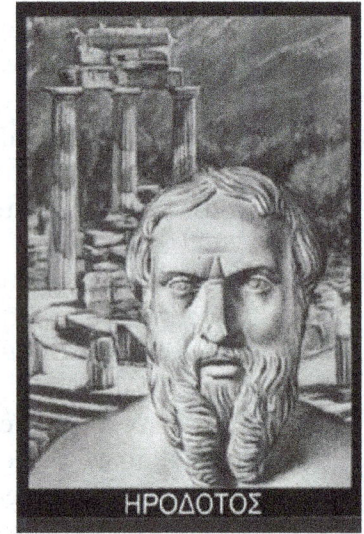

You can even go further back and look at Herodotus. This is a story that I've told before, but I think it's very, very interesting:

Herodotus was the father of history, he's the first person that started chronicling things down and giving us a historical record.

He went all over the world and chronicled very important things. That's the only reason we have records of a lot of these things and these wars and these meetings between different dignitaries of different countries.

One of them was between a diplomat from the Persian Empire who went down to Ethiopia after Persia had taken over Egypt. And they were talking getting to know their new neighbors... and the King of Ethiopia asked the Persian emissary "What do your people eat, and how long do your people normally live?"

So the Persian guy described growing crops and making bread out of wheat, and he said that "Our people would normally live around 70 years." And the king of Ethiopia sort of laughed at him and said

"Well, no wonder you live such short lives if all you eat is dirt! We exclusively eat boiled meat from our livestock and we only drink the milk from our livestock - and our people live 120 years and sometimes more!"

That might sound a bit far-fetched. In fact, in the Australian Aborigines and the Inuits, the Massai and Native Americans and other such cultures that just ate meat, they actually talk about this longevity

Dr. Salisbury chronicles that in his book in the 1800s: He lived with the Native Americans. They said these [older] people were hail and hearty, running around the pack on their back, following the buffalo herds day in and day out, at 105, 110, 115 years old. They're not sitting in a nursing home, turning to dust for 40 years! They're active adults in good health.

All of this sounds very far-fetched to modern day people, who start breaking down in their 30s and just start dying and getting obese and heart disease and other sort of issues very early on in life.

But we've actually known for about 20 years now, as geneticists, that chromosomally humans are designed to live about 120 years. On average! Meaning that if you just stay out of your own way and don't mess up, you should make it to 120 years without doing anything special. Okay?

So why are we dying in our 60s and 70s, on average? That is literally middle aged! And yet, this is the common theme around the world, is, that our bodies just start breaking down after 30, they really start breaking down after 40...

Then you get into your *older age,* in your 50s... and we call this a senior citizen. We get senior citizen discounts at 55 in some places. That's less than middle age. That should be in the prime of your adulthood - and yet, it's not. Yet, we're breaking down and getting more and more sick. Unless you don't eat things that cause harm.

Metabolically:

In biochemistry, we talk about a *fed state* versus a *fasting state*. So a fed state traditionally would mean: If you eat, this is what your biochemistry looks like. And when you stop eating, your biochemistry switches into a different program in order to keep you alive and maintain things - while you don't have any incoming food.

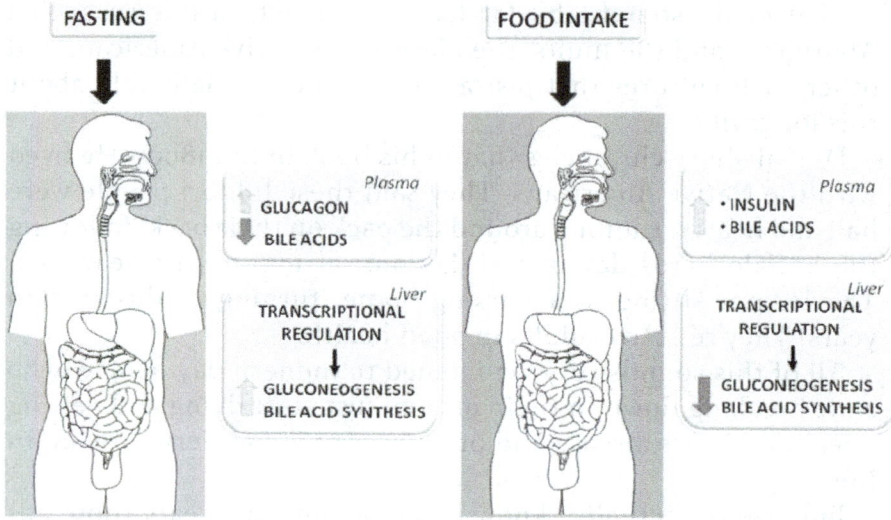

I think that's completely wrong! I think that our so-called fasting state is actually our *primary* metabolic state! This is the primary metabolic state of basically all animals in the wild.

We have studies on this, going back to 1981 with wolves. They said "Well, you have to eat carbs to burn carbs", that was the thought.

But wolves don't carb-load before they chase caribou for 10 hours! Do they have blood sugar, do they have muscle and liver glycogen? They found out: Yes, they actually do... and it's rock solid, it does not change. No matter what they're doing, it's basically the same. There's just subtle variations.

But they are in this so-called fasted state and that allows their body to mobilize energy and nutrition from their fat stores.

That's our primary metabolic state as well: When you eat carbohydrates, it raises your insulin. Insulin basically shuts down your metabolism, and it slows your metabolism! Your basal metabolic rate drops on average by 300 kilocalories a day. So on average, you will burn 300 less kilocalories, food calories, a day when eating carbohydrate-containing foods!

So if you have 2000 calories with carbs in the mix, and 2000 calories without carbs in the mix, you will burn 300 more food calories a day without the carbs. And so this whole *calorie-in calorie-out* thing gets a bit more complicated.

Because it's not as simple as people think... what you eat determines what your output will be, what your metabolic rate will be! So it's not as easy to figure out exactly what your metabolic rate is, it's not as easy to figure out exactly how much energy your body is producing.

These are also complex organic chemicals, they obviously have complex organic chemical interactions with your body.

So a carbohydrate is a lot more than a calorie. As are proteins, as are fats. There are many different kinds of fats, there are many different kinds of carbohydrates. There are many different kind of proteins. And these have different chemical effects in your body, they do different things in your body. They're used for different things in your body.

You cannot just look at them as a caloric source because that is not what they are! They fundamentally change your body... and insulin especially is problematic because it will, again, slow your metabolism. It stops energy from coming out of your cells, it forces energy into cells and stops energy from coming out of cells.

Insulin blocks proteolysis, it blocks lipolysis. Without lipolysis, you cannot break down your fat stores to make energy, to go through gluconeogenesis and make blood sugar and glycogen, and to make ketones to run your body and your brain. So you shut down that whole process.

But insulin also does something more insidious:

It blocks a hormone called leptin - which is secreted from your fat stores - and tells your brain how much energy you have. Leptin is like a running gas gauge on how much energy your body has.

And so your brain looks at that, goes "Oh, we got plenty of energy, we don't need to eat."

Or: It gets blocked by insulin... and fructose, by the way. Now your brain can't see its leptin, it thinks you're starving to death. Your blood sugar is dropping because your insulin is up which forces your blood sugar to go down. And your brain sends out a panic signal that says "If you don't eat now, you will die!"

This is why multiple times a day, people think that they're dying and they need to eat constant amounts of food.

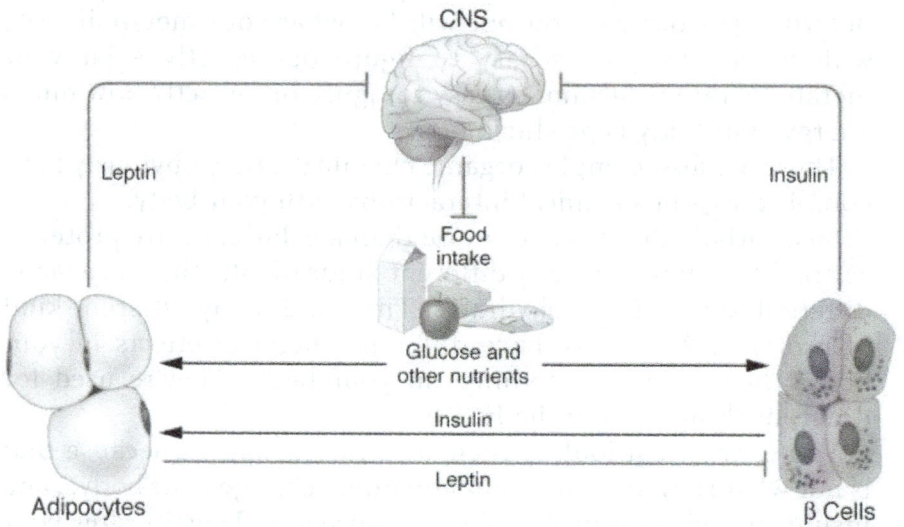

This is a just a depiction of that leptin-insulin cycle and it gets disrupted by carbohydrates.

So when you eat carbohydrates, your blood sugar necessarily goes up. Well, this is not a good thing. People think it's "Oh I'm getting more energy, that helps me." No, it doesn't, actually.

High blood sugar is actually damaging to your body! This is because glucose molecules can physically fuse to other molecules and damage them, to make them act abnormally, pathologically, or just not at all. It's called *glycation*.

Fructose is actually worse than this, it does more of this in your body.

So in a defensive mechanism, your insulin goes up, right? Because this high blood sugar, chronic high blood sugar, this is actually what kills diabetics, this is what breaks them down! This is, again, that toxicity model in full view. Where you're eating something and this is damaging your body.

And we've had... I think, over 100 years of scientific literature showing that a ketogenic diet is very efficacious for treating diabetics.

This is a poison relationship! You're removing carbohydrates, you're removing sugar, you're removing alcohol. You're removing the precipitous factors that cause these diseases, like diabetes.

Cancer is another major one. Otto Warburg described in in the 1930s and 40s - and he actually won the Nobel Prize in medicine for his work in cancer biology - that cancer cells feed on glucose. In fact, they need about 400 times the amount of glucose that normal cells do! This is because their mitochondria are damaged. Otto Warburg showed that if you have healthy mitochondria, *you cannot get cancer.*

This is something that's been reiterated and actually proven true, by the work of such people as **Professor Thomas Seyfried** of Boston College, who I've had on my podcast as well. I encourage everyone to go look at his stuff.

He wrote a book called **Cancer as a metabolic disease**. It is! If you look at the cancer biology... and this is in textbooks, this is not a fringe opinion, this is hard biochemistry.

If your mitochondria work properly, they stay in oxidative phosphorylation. That uses oxygen to make an abundant amount of ATP.

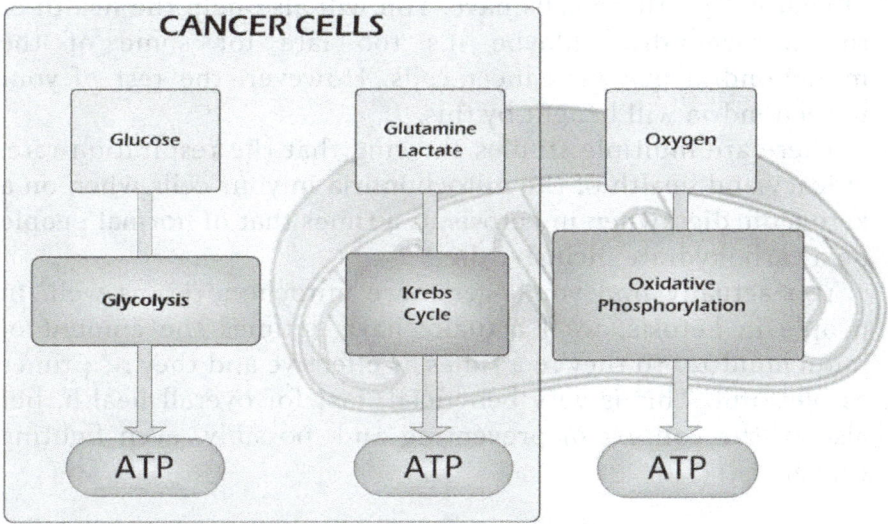

When your mitochondria get damaged, they stop being able to do that and they go into a fermentative process. Then it actually takes a lot more glucose to make ATP. Because you're getting 36 ATP from oxidative phosphorylation, but you're only getting 2 ATP when you're doing it anaerobically.

So then this produces lactate as well, which is that burning in your muscles when you're working out. That sort of burn, the feel of burn, that's that lactic acid buildup that actually hurts.

Cancer cells produce a lot of lactate, and this actually makes sort of a swamp around them, that makes it hard for other cells to get in close and try to attack them.

This is something, too, that that Professor Seyfried has shown. That:

If you go on a ketogenic diet, this actually starves out your cancer cells! It limits the supply of glucose to those cancer cells, which again, need 400 times the amount of glucose that other cells do. Because they're much less efficient at making it, and they're trying to grow just out of control.

The reason they're trying to grow out of control, by the way, is because the mitochondria are actually what regulate cell growth. So when the mitochondria get damaged and they can't do their job, they can't control their growth - and so we get out of control growth, which is what cancer is.

So when you go on a ketogenic diet, you will limit the amount of energy that those cells have. You will also help the health of the mitochondria. Maybe it's too late for some of the mitochondria in your cancer cells. However, the rest of your mitochondria will benefit by this.

There are multiple studies showing that the respiration rate, efficacy and health of the mitochondria in your cells when on a ketogenic diet, when in ketosis, is 4 times that of normal people on a carbohydrate inclusive diet!

You actually find you'll get more mitochondria, as well. In people in ketosis, we'll actually have 4 times the amount of mitochondria. So they're 4 times as effective and they're 4 times as plentiful. This is very beneficial, just for overall health, but also in the context of preventing and, possibly, even fighting cancer.

This is something that's actually been picked up by other medical groups, such as *Paleomedicina* in Hungary. Which have been using at least a ketogenic, if not a carnivore diet, for people for well over 10 years. With cancer, with Crohn's, with other metabolic diseases - and they're having fantastic results.

This is becoming recognized in America as well, and even Cedars-Sinai has started instituting metabolic treatments for cancer, too. Which includes nutritional ketosis as a driving force in that treatment.

Again, going back to the fact that this all stems from plants being toxic...

Plants are trying to kill you:
The reason I say plants are trying to kill you, it's not that they're necessarily out to get you per se. I don't think they really care one way or the other if you're around... unless they want you to go down and become fertilizer for them.

But this all stems from when I was taking cancer biology 20 years ago at the University of Washington in Seattle. We learned on day one how toxic plants were. This is something that we actually learned before that...

I remember in 7th grade biology, we learned that plants and animals were in an evolutionary arms race: Plants becoming more and more toxic, so less and less animals could eat them, so they could survive and thrive. Otherwise, they'd go extinct!

And then animals who eat plants, eating a specific plant, becoming more and more adapted to that specific plant, and coevolving with that plant. To become more resistant to being able to break down those poisons into safe by-products, so that they can survive and thrive.

So if you're not part of that evolutionary arms race, you're going to start losing. Right? Because you're not going to have those built-in defenses against these poisons. And we were looking at this from a cancer perspective.

We were taught that

- Brussels sprouts had 136 known human carcinogens in them and
- Mushrooms had over 100.
- Spinach, lettuce, celery, cabbage, cucumber, broccoli, you name it...

...they all had 60, 80 or over 100 known human carcinogens in them

and they were quite abundant!

We know from the work of Professor Bruce Ames from Berkeley: In 1989, he published a paper that actually compared the plant toxins already existing in the vegetables that we eat - comparing them to the pesticides we spray on them.

Because we say "Well, if you grow it in your own garden, then it's okay! Get away from these pesticides!" No, no. It's the plant that was the problem in the first place! They were saying this in the 80s, too "We got to get rid of these pesticides, we've got to get rid of them!"

So he did a study and said "Okay. Well, what are we looking at here?" He found that there were 42 different poisons identified in these plants, 20 of which were shown to be carcinogenic in the lab and... Obviously, we found many, many more just in the 12 years in between when I took cancer biology and learned all this.

But back in 1989, they found that of those 42 chemicals, they were 10,000 times more abundant by weight than the pesticides we sprayed on these plants. Okay? So the spinach was worse than the pesticides. It was 10,000 times more abundant, and the naturally occurring poisons were orders of magnitude times more likely to cause cancer than the pesticides we spray on them.

This is why we still have pesticides! This is why they weren't outlawed and banned. Because they showed scientifically that the plant is worse than the pesticide! So if you're going to eat the plant, you probably don't need to worry about the pesticide.

Now, that's not to say that pesticides are good for you. Especially things like Roundup and all these other things. No, they are not. But the plants aren't either, that's the whole point. And so, we were quite taken aback by this, as you could imagine.

I thought that our teacher must be joking, everyone thought he must be joking. Everyone was looking around, thrashing their heads around wildly, cackling in the corner, trying to keep it together - because this was obviously a joke. It was not a joke!

He was not joking, it finally dawned on us. I remember thinking like "Okay, he's serious. But... but... vegetables are still good for you, though? Right?" And he must have just read our minds, because he looked at us and just said:

> I don't eat salad. I don't eat vegetables. I don't let my kids eat vegetables. Plants are trying to kill you!

So I said "All right, screw plants" - and I just stopped eating plants from that day on. That's why I've been doing carnivore, inadvertently, for about 22 years now.

Because I learned that plants were toxic, they don't want you to eat them. If you start eating them, they are going to make it hard on you. And they're going to make you feel like crap and they're going to try to kill you.

We know this intuitively: If you get lost in the woods, you can't just eat any random plant. Most plants will kill you, or at least make you very, very sick. These are inedible plants, right? So why do we think that the so-called edible plants are just from the Garden of Eden and just couldn't be better for you?

In fact, they're not. They're actually quite harmful as well. It's just they're not as harmful as a hemlock.

Let's look at some of these things:

There are a lot of different **toxins** that exist in these. These are things like cassava, which as a caloric source is the third most important source in the third world.

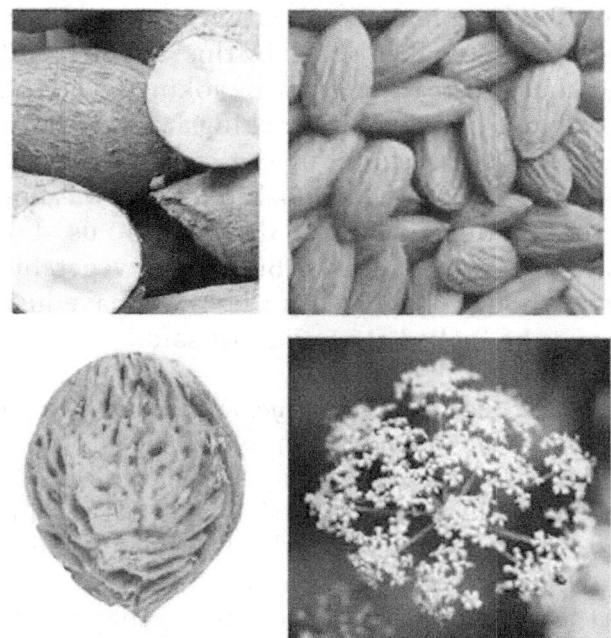

You have almonds which contain cyanide. There's 2500 different cyanide containing plants that we know of, and they go by crush receptors. Or pressure spots.

The toxins don't just exist free floating in the seed or the nut, but when they're crushed, then the cyanide is released. Well, what is crushing? That's something chewing and masticating that thing - and the plant goes "Right, you're going to eat me, I'm going to poison you!" So it releases this poison pill, it says "I'm going to take you down with me!"

You look at that pip, that's like a peach pip. When you open that up, you crack that stone open, it looks like a shriveled almond. It's actually called a bitter almond. And this has enough cyanide in it, that when chewed, to release the cyanide, one or two of those can kill you. Okay?

Almonds, it takes around a pound or two, depending on the almonds because they have varying amounts of cyanide in them... it takes a pound or two of almonds to get a lethal dose of cyanide. I have sat down and just hand balled half a pound of almonds from a Costco bag of these things before. That's potentially half a lethal dose! You know, I'm a bigger person, so maybe it wasn't half of a lethal dose for me. But that that is absolutely terrifying! We just sell this in stores where kids can get them, that is insane.

And while you may not die eating these amounts of cyanide, they can actually cause a lot of harm to your body. It can cause damage your thyroid, damage to your brain as well. They're neurotoxic.

Let's look at some of these in specificity, let's look at hormone disruptors: There are things like called **phytoestrogens**. These are very commonly produced throughout the plant kingdom. Most notably in soy, about 3 ounces of soy have over a million nanograms of phytoestrogens in them.

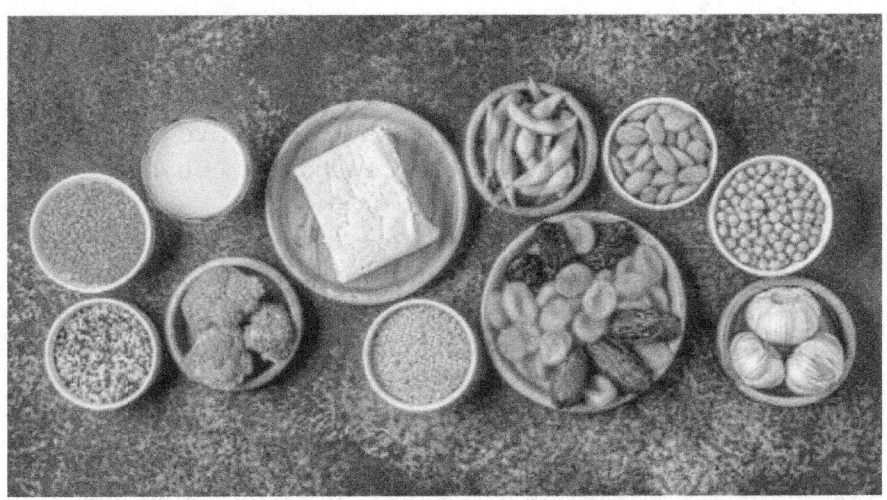

Put that in comparison to a fertile woman, who makes about 180,000 nanograms a day. So this is multiple times what they would make in a day, just in those three ounces. The birth control pill, depending on the birth control pill, would have 35,000 nanograms of estrogen.

They say "What about beef? You have this hormone treated animals, they have all these hormones in them!" Right... three ounces of lean beef, that is hormone treated - given growth hormone supplementation throughout their life - has about 4 nanograms of estrogen in it. So not the same thing, not on the same scale whatsoever.

There are other things that increase testosterone, but also things that block and suppress testosterone. Block and suppress estrogen. Even just carbohydrates will suppress the conversion of testosterone into estrogen in women.

Women don't just make estrogen, they actually make testosterone first and then that testosterone is converted into estrogen in the ovaries. But high insulin levels will actually block that conversion. So just that high insulin is actually causing harm throughout your body.

It's blocking leptin, it's blocking conversion of your hormones, it's doing a lot of damage throughout your body. So that's, again, another way that we can tell that that's not our normal biochemical state, because we're actually screwing up our biochemistry.

This is where PCOS comes into play, when women are eating a lot of carbohydrates. Some will be more sensitive than others. However, for all of them, when they're eating carbohydrates their insulin will go up.

That will block the conversion of testosterone into estrogen - and so they will necessarily have more testosterone than their body wants, and they'll have less estrogen than their body wants. Or needs. This disrupts our hormones quite significantly. And there are other factors that that do that as well.

Then you have **nutrient blockers:** These are different substrates and substances that that block absorption or digestion. We already talked about fiber, how that makes a physical barrier between your enzymes and the food. So it can't break down the food into amino acids in the first place, or into shorter portioned out fatty acids.

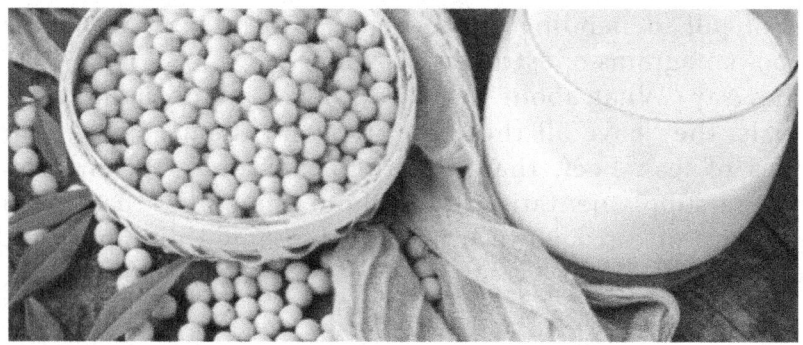

Then, once those things are broken down, this is a physical barrier from those nutrients getting to the border of your intestine, to be drawn into the cell in the first place. So those get blocked and taken out.

But more specifically, just looking at soy and wheat: They make a protease inhibitor. Protease is released from your pancreas to break down protein, as it sounds. Something like -*ase*, that means it's breaking something down. A protease inhibitor stops that, okay?

So soy and wheat have **protease inhibitors**, that block protease from breaking down our protein. This gets into bioavailability of plants as well.

The protein that's available, or that exists, in plants are not available necessarily. Gluten makes up 80% of the protein in
40
wheat - gluten cannot be used as protein. Your body cannot break it down, it cannot absorb it, it cannot use it as protein. Period!

And? It has protease inhibitors! So what little is left of the protein in wheat, that your body can actually do anything with, now your body can't do anything with it because it's blocking the breakdown of it.

But also: If you are eating meat, with its very bioavailable proteins and fats... when you're eating it with wheat - like in a sandwich, or you put some croutons or breaded chicken – what you're doing there is, you're going to block protease from breaking down the meat as well.

You're actually going to, again, waste nutrients, waste nutrition. And that cannot be beneficial to our survival. So that cannot be what we're supposed to eat.

Soy does the same thing, soy has protease inhibitors as well. And there are many, many others and many other examples of these nutrient blockers.

Photosensitivity: This is one that not many people know about. But there are many plants that actually cause us to be much more sensitive to sunlight. With others, it's just increased inflammation, increased damage.

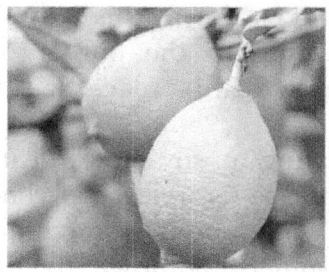 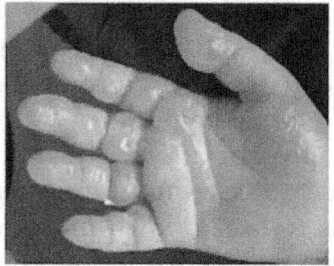

So we get some damage from the sun and that increases that inflammatory response and damage, so our sunburns are worse. They hurt worse, they damage our DNA worse, we get worse peeling and a higher risk for skin cancers.

But specifically, the things that cause you to be much more sensitive to UV light are things like limes. There's oils in limes... and remember, a lime is an unripe fruit. Now, the plant may or may not want you to eat that fruit.

It mostly wants other animals to eat that fruit! Most fruit will kill you. Most berries will kill you.

But there are some that may not be as toxic, or contain fructose. These generally have much less defense chemicals in them and that's why we find fructose to be sweet. Because we recognize that as safe, and so it's like "Okay, this can give me a quick hit of energy and that will make me survive!"

But fructose in and of itself will cause a lot of harm. As a fact, its breakdown is like alcohol and causes the same damages as alcohol.

So lime's being an unripe fruit, its seed is not ready to be eaten. It has defenses, it has defense chemicals. This is where like green tomatoes come in, these are traditionally known to be toxic, and you don't eat them. You want them to be vine ripened.

In a lime, it secretes oils on the outside and if you touch them, if you handle them, they will soak in your skin and it causes you to be very, very sensitive to sunlight.

There's actually documented cases of people getting second degree burns just from handling limes in the sun. That actually happened to my younger brother when we were kids in southern California:

We had a lime tree and he was out there, sort of picking limes and playing around - and all of a sudden came in and he had these massive red welts and wheels all over his body. We thought that he must have be having a sensitizing reaction, and the next time he would get anaphylaxis and he'd be dead!

And so it was like "Okay, keep that kid away from limes and lime trees." He hasn't eaten and used lime since then and hasn't had any sort of problem. So that is really looking back what happened.

There are other things that will also do the same. There's a thing called celery dermatitis, where people who handle a lot of celery, pick celery, eat a lot of celery, will get very, very sensitive. They'll have to wear hats and long sleeve shirts, even gloves and put sun cream on everywhere, because they will just get absolutely scorched in the sun.

This also goes into why we generally don't see too many tanned vegans, a lot of them will get burned and torn up. I do fine, I don't get burnt in the sun.

You talk to any carnivore who has been doing this for a while, they're amazed - they don't get burns in the sun! You might get red, that's just blood going to the skin, but that just turns into a tan later. You're not really going to peel or damage your skin unless you really overdo it.

We talked about the **cyanogenic** properties of different plants, there's 2500 different plants that use cyanide as a defense. This is very clearly designed to stop animals from eating them because it has that crush effect. They only release the cyanide when they are crushed.

Then you have **nightshades:** These are potatoes, tomatoes, eggplants, peppers. These have been known for thousands of years to be just an entire class of plants that you just don't go near.

The Europeans, going back millennia, knew that you don't touch nightshades. They could tell when they went to the new world, they'd say "Oh, that these are nightshades don't eat them!"

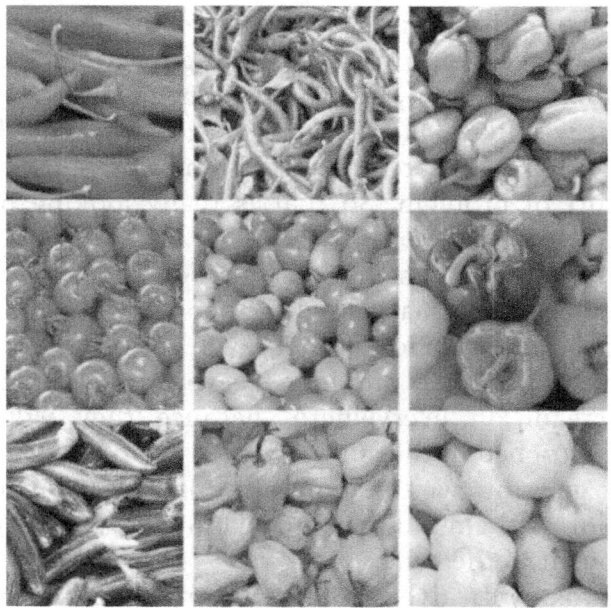

They brought them back as curiosities "What a strange looking plant, look at what we brought back from this strange new land!" It was seen that the some of the natives were eating these things, but they were doing it in very specific ways.

They were taking the tomatoes, they were blanching them, they were taking the peel off, they were taking the seeds out. They were only eating the pulp - and that's actually what traditional tomato sauces were made out of, just that pulp of vine ripened tomatoes.

They would peel the skin of a potato... up until very recently, it's only been within my lifetime that people said "No, no, you don't want to peel these plants and these vegetables, that's where all the nutrients are! That's where all the vitamins are!"

Yeah, okay - it's also where all the poison is! That's their barrier of protection, that stops insects from eating into them and eating this part of the plant that they don't want eaten.

Then we got **gluten**.

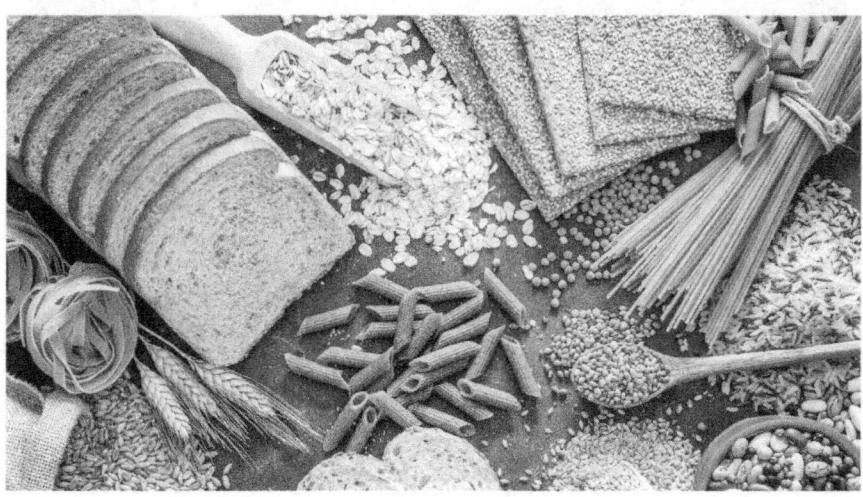

Again, this is a protein but it is not possible to be used as protein. It also causes a lot of harm. It actually causes leaky gut, which is the breakdown of those tight junctions in between your intestinal cells, in the intestinal wall.

This allows chemicals such as lectins and other things, even bacteria, to get into your system and getting into your body, when normally they would not do that. They would stay out by that barrier protection, just like your skin stops bugs and weird things from getting into your body. Your gut lining does the same thing. So really, the lumen of your intestine, that's the outside world. Your body's not letting that in, unless you're eating things like gluten and that breaks down that barrier protection, so now these things can get into your body and cause harm.

This is where lectins come in: I mean, there's a whole book written about this in 2019 by Dr. Gundry, who showed just how harmful lectins are.

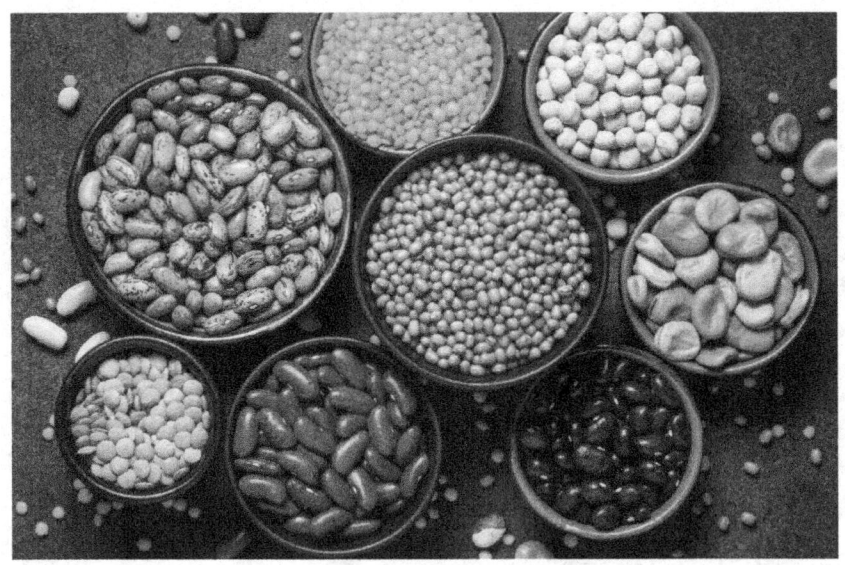

Things like kidney beans which are very normal things to eat. When you don't process them properly, when you don't soak them in water and then boil them for at least 10 minutes, those lectins can make you very, very sick.

Even then, they're not done away with, they're not perfectly disabled. They still cause harm in your body and of course your heat treatment isn't going to take care of all the plant toxins out there.

Lectins specifically will get into your body through these tight junctions. They've actually been indicated to be a causative factor in autoimmune issues! The body makes antibodies towards these lectins because these are foreign molecules, your body does not want them in your body. So it fights them, makes these antibodies to go out and attack these things.

Well, there's something called molecular mimicry, where some protein or something on one of your cells may be similar enough to one of these lectins (or a bacteria or virus that your body's fighting off) that these antibodies stick to them.

Because they don't have a mind of their own, they're just acting chemically. And if they can bind to something chemically, they will bind to that. It's just a chemical reaction. So by molecular mimicry, all of a sudden your body has started attacking your own body, that's an autoimmune disease.

Autoimmune, meaning your body is attacking itself. But it's not attacking itself, it's attacking these lectins. And when you remove those lectins from your diet, your body stops making antibodies towards those lectins - and then there's no spillover effect from those antibodies to your body.

This is why nearly every single autoimmune disease that I've ever seen in people, who went on a carnivore diet will significantly improve, if not completely resolve within a few months. I have yet to see someone with Crohn's or ulcerative colitis go on a carnivore diet, usually red meat and water diet - and not completely reverse their disease within 3 months. On biopsy!

So when these guys get biopsied at 3 months, there's no sign of disease. I have yet to see a single case in that that didn't happen.

Rheumatoid arthritis as well, that just goes away. People will get much better within the first few weeks already - and then even on biopsy, they'll find that there's no sign of disease after a few months.

Hashimoto's takes a little bit longer. You usually see that take about 9 months to a year... or maybe just still lingering on a little bit. But it significantly improves.

Again, with Dr. Salisbury, he was showing that you could reverse rheumatoid arthritis, Crohn's and ulcerative colitis, back in the 1800s, by putting people on a pure red meat and water diet. This was something that was well known and documented in the peer-reviewed medical literature, going back to the 1800s.

And yet, no one knows about it. Why is that?

Then, there are other things that'll just kill you straight out. We talked about the inedible plants, like North American water hemlock:

This blocks the GABBA receptors in your brain that basically calm down your brain cells. When your brain cells get too stimulated, overstimulated and out of control, they all start firing at once - and this is called a seizure. Okay? Those can be quite dangerous, they actually damage your brain directly.

They also can make you fall over and crack your head, if you don't stop having a seizure. You can die, or... you will die, if you don't stop.

Hemlock blocks the GABBA receptor. All the medications that we use to stop seizures, they basically all work on that GABBA receptor, and this is blocking that. So it doesn't matter how much medication and drugs you give these people, they're going to die of seizures within one to two minutes. And you're never going to get to them fast enough to stop it anyway, even if it does have some effect.

This is a very well developed, well catalogued and described phenomenon in botany. Going back thousands of years, that plants use harmful chemicals to stop animals and insects from eating them.

Okay, so in summary: This really shows that we are **obligate carnivores** - with one optimal diet!

We are therefore 'Obligate' Carnivores with ONE Optimal diet...

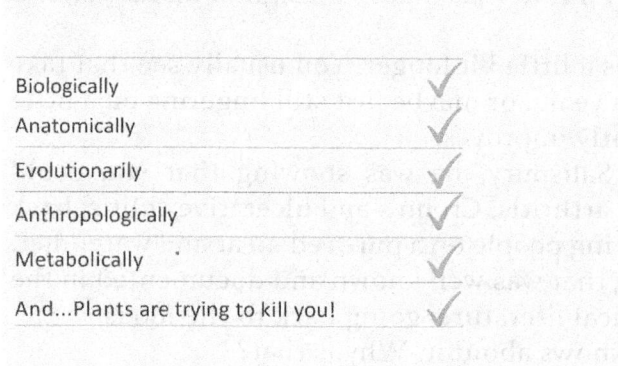
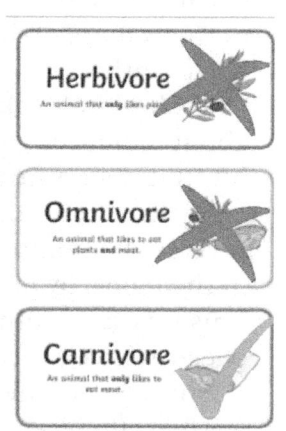

Biologically ✓
Anatomically ✓
Evolutionarily ✓
Anthropologically ✓
Metabolically ✓
And...Plants are trying to kill you! ✓

We are obligated to eat meat! We cannot thrive and survive on anything else, okay? While we can survive eating other things, we're not going to thrive. That's not going to be optimal for us.

I know, some people say "Well, everyone's different and maybe one person does better with an omnivore diet, maybe someone does better with a vegetarian diet. Maybe someone does better with meat based diet. Everyone's different."

That is nonsense. That is someone who has not thought about this for literally one second. And when I hear doctors say this sort of thing, I really get a bit miffed - because these are people that are supposedly biologists. But I guess everyone forgot their biology lesson and forgot to actually just look out in nature.

Anytime someone says this, I ask them... I've asked doctors this, I've asked other people this, people that have made this ridiculous comment. I ask:

"Name one example of two members of the same species who have different optimal diets! Okay? It does not exist!" People say "Well, is this good for women as well as for men? What about during pregnancy, what about kids?" The answer is just *Yes!*

It doesn't matter what condition you are in, what stage of life you are. Whatever. We are humans. We are homo sapien sapiens. If we had a different optimal diet between two people, those two people would be different species of people. And yet, they're not.

We don't have different species of people, anymore. We don't even have homo neanderthalis anymore, we just have homo sapiens... and Neanderthals were carnivores as well.

You have to be actually quite divergent, you can't even be a close relative and have a very different diet. All right?

So
- Biologically
- Anatomically
- Evolutionarily
- Anthropologically and
- Metabolically

we can show that humans are carnivores. That is just the kind of animal that we are, and that eating meat is our optimal diet. And for no less reason than plants use defense chemicals because they don't want to die.

If it's you or them, they will make sure it's you, okay? Because it's *killer / be killed* out in the wild, even for plants. As well as animals.

I've never seen a cave painting of a salad, either.

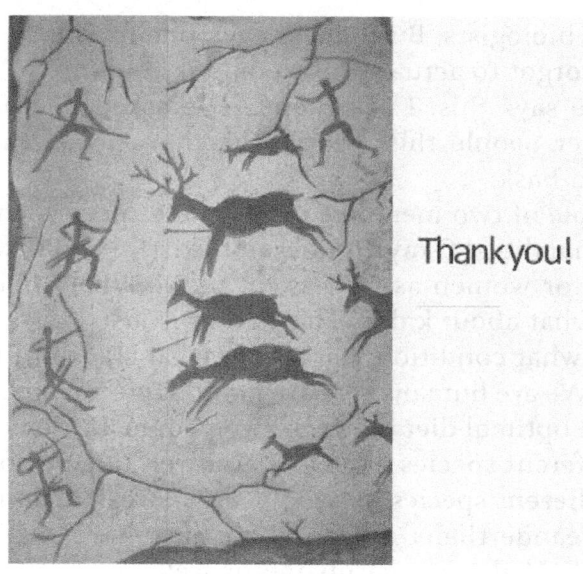

Thank you!

I hope you guys liked that talk. I have some of my references here that people can take a look at:

References

Anatomically

Neil Roach, Brian Richmond: *Clavicle length, throwing performance and*
the reconstruction of the Homo erectus shoulder
November 2014, Journal of Human Evolution, 80.
DOI:10.1016/j.jhevol.2014.09.004

Anatomically - Eyes

Arizona Retina Project
https://azretina.sites.arizona.edu/node/601

Evolutionarily

Tools-Discover Magazine: *The Evolutionary Timeline Retooled*
https://www.discovermagazine.com/environment/the-evolutionarytimeline-retooled

Ice Ages - Smithsonian Magazine: *Scientists Project Precisely How Cold the Last Ice Age Was*

Stable Isotopes - Richard's MP *(2000) Archeolog Sci 27 (1): 1-3* and Michael Eades *'Paleopathology and the Origins of the low carb diet'*, Low Carb Down Under conference 2020,
https://www.researchgate.net/publication/331735735 Stable isotopes reveal patterns of diet and mobility in the last Neandertals and first modern humans in Europe

Statue of Hemiunu - http://giza.fas.harvard.edu/objects/54706/full/

Israeli Study: *American Journal of Physical Anthropology (Yearbook of Physical Anthropology article)*,

Dr. Miki Ben-Dor and Prof. Ran Barkai of the Jacob M. Alkov Department of Archaeology at Tel Aviv University
https://onlinelibrary.wiley.com/doi/10.1002/ajpa.24247

Teeth and Jaw records - The agricultural revolution as environmental catastrophe: Implications for health and lifestyle in the Holocene, Science Direct, Vol 150.

Harvard crimson: dental health of Inuit carnivores https://www.thecrimson.com/article/1929/1/29/esquimo-teeth-provehealth-of-meat/#.W53lycLPrQc.twitter

Brain size - *When and Why did Human Brains Decrease in Size? A New Change-Point analysis and Insights from Brain Evolution* in Ants, Frontier in Ecology and Evolution

Anthropologically

Fat of the Land - Vilhjalmur Stefansson

Nutrition and Physical Degeneration - Weston Price

The French Explorers and the Aboriginal Australians 1772-1839 - Colin Dyer

Metabolically

Metabolic Theory of Cancer https://www.tieospharma.com/science

Ketogenic diets and cancer treatment
https://www.ncbi.nlm.nih.gov/pmc/articles/PMC6375425/

Dr Thomas Seyfried *Cancer, mitochondria, and ketogenic diet and fasting in cancer treatment* https://youtu.be/PuG5XZSR4vs

Keto and glutamine, GBM treatment Seyfried
https://www.nature.com/articles/s42003-019-0455-x Cancer causing polyunsaturated fat (Mitochondria effect)

https://www.sciencedirect.com/science/article/pii/S2213231714001359

Plants are trying to kill you

Natural pesticides in vegetables
http://www.garfield.library.upenn.edu/papers/vethumtoxicology31(6)p589y1989.html

https://www.the-scientist.com/?articles.view/articleNo/10489/title/Man-Made-and-Natural-Carcinogens--Putting-TheRisks-In-Perspective/
Science (244:755-7, May 19,1989)

WHO Natural Plant Toxins https://www.who.int/news-room/factsheets/detail/natural-toxins-in-food?fbclid=lwAR2j8SyhGBJzPLilro51J4BLNRKKVyGaN344Um9ACLAC-Q13jckUYSe7DY

175 countries: More meat, more health and longevity
https://www.researchgate.net/publication/358754564 *Total Meat Intake is Associated with Life Expectancy A Cross- Sectional Data Analysis of 175 Contemporary Populations*

Harvard Carnivore study, 2000+ people
https://academic.oup.com/cdn/advancearticle/doi/10.1093/cdn/nzab133/6415894

Journal of the American College of Cardiology - Volume 76, Issue 7, 18 August 2020, Pages 844-857

Autism vegetarians/vegans (carnitine deficiency)
https://www.sciencedirect.com/science/article/pii/S2211124716000085

Sugar industry cover up, JAMA 2015
https://jamanetwork.com/journals/jamainternalmedicine/articleabstract/2548255

Red meat doesn't increase risk of colon cancer or all cause mortality
https://www.mdpi.com/2072-6643/13/1/32

Chapter 2

Carnivore for Beginners. How to start a Carnivore Diet. With tips, tricks and common pitfalls

Hey guys, Dr. Chaffee here! I just wanted to do a quick little video on how to start carnivore. Just some of the tips and tricks that I tell people, like my patients, friends or people, that are trying to start carnivore.

It's quite simple: You're just eating meat and drinking water - and that's it, okay?

- You can salt to taste
- Eat fatty meat, fats are very important
- You can eat organs if you want, but you don't have to. And
- You don't want to get too many organs because you can actually get hypervitaminosis

People talk about how nutrient dense organs are, and that's true. But that can also be a problem because they're much more nutrient dense than muscle meat, which has everything you need.

By definition, it's going to have a little too much. So if you're eating this stuff out of proportion of the animal...

Remember: How many hundreds of pounds of muscle and fat a cow is going to have, to every one pound of liver - it's not going to be a lot of liver every day, okay?

So a bit of liver, a bit of organs, is totally fine. Don't overdo it. And you don't have to have any if you don't want it then. You just don't eat them. I don't eat them and I've been doing this for years. The most important thing is really about *what not to eat as*, opposed to what to eat. We know what we need to eat: Meat! Drink water, get the fat. But it's much more important what not to eat.

My hard rules are:
- No Plants
- No sugars
- Nothing artificial, and
- that goes for sauces, seasonings and drinks as well

So it's just animal meat and *not* animal products.

"Oh honey, that's an animal product!" Well, it's actually bee vomit... they're just vomiting up concentrated nectar - which comes from a plant! But it's also a kind of sugar. And there's more fructose in honey than high fructose corn syrup, and this is bad.

People may argue that in the form of honey, fructose is actually good for you. But they have absolutely no evidence whatsoever, to back that up with. All of the best evidence that we have is that fructose causes harm, so I would avoid that at all costs.

So, some of the pitfalls that people cut through:

A lot of people come to carnivore because they want to lose some weight, they want to address medical issues, or maybe they just want to optimize their health.

But they're used to having to eat in a disordered fashion, with Western diets, vegetarian or vegan diets - where you have to worry about portion control and calorie counting, intermittent fasting, all these things.

You don't need to do this. You just eat fatty meat when you're hungry, and you eat until you're satiated. So you eat *until it stops tasting good!*

If meat doesn't taste good, it means you're not hungry. But if it does taste good, you are, so you should listen to that. If the meat tastes good, eat it. Eat it until it doesn't really taste good anymore, then just stop. Let your body be the judge of what you need.

If you're not eating carbohydrates, you can actually listen to your hunger signals. It's the carbohydrates that negatively rearrange your hormonal signaling pathways, to make you think you're hungry when you're not.

So if you're not eating carbohydrates, you're not going to be feeling hungry when you're not actually hungry. You actually have to relearn your hunger signals.

That's something to watch out for as well, because some people can undereat! When I was first doing this, I definitely underate because I didn't realize that fact... that was 20 years ago or so.

But I wasn't eating enough because I never felt hungry! But then I relearned my hunger signals and realized what hunger actually felt like.

Fasting: You don't need to fast, you don't need to intermittent fast.

These things can be helpful, especially when eating a Western diet. But all the studies show a benefit, as compared to a western diet - but not really a benefit when compared to what they call a *fasting mimicking diet* (which is a ketogenic diet).

So the majority of the benefits are coming from just getting into the metabolic state, which is our so-called *fasting state* – that's what we call it in biochemistry.

But I argue that this is our primary metabolic state. In this fasting metabolic state, all of our heavy machinery comes to bear, this is the metabolic state of animals in the wild. Including humans, because humans are eating meat.

Exercise: People think "Well, if I'm eating all this fatty meat, that's going to make me gain a lot of fat, unless I exercise a lot!" That's actually not true. You don't have to.

I don't exercise a lot, but I do look like I work out... but I actually don't have time to work out that much, because I'm just swamped at the hospital with everything I'm doing.

I love to work out! I absolutely get a lot out of it and I really enjoy it. I'm actually going to the gym after this, but you don't have to do that to achieve optimal health.

The food is the optimal health, you're putting in the optimal fuel and that will optimize your workouts as well, and you'll get a lot more out of them when you do workout. You'll get a lot of benefit from working out.

You don't have to eat certain meats only: You can eat fish or chicken - all these sorts of things, any meat that you enjoy is fine. Any meat that tastes good, that makes you feel good and that you can afford is fine.

But: Some people do have different sensitivities, especially people with autoimmune issues.

Sometimes they have to actually stay more towards at the beef / grass-fed beef side of things. The reason is that even chicken, pork or even egg whites can actually cause problem when they're still healing. Because they're still very sensitive to these things.

But if you're not one of those people, you can have eggs, have chicken, have whatever you want.

> Really, all this comes down to is:
> **Don't make it complicated!**
> Eat meat, drink water, be happy!

Get on with your life. You just eat until you're full and enjoy the rest of your day.

This way of eating is going to save you huge amounts of time, so don't overthink it. You don't have to track every little calorie, you don't have to track every little macro. Just eat what tastes good, stop when it stops tasting good - and your body will do the rest!

Your body knows what it's doing. If you need a calculator to figure out what to eat, you're eating the wrong thing. Because nature is natural. It just happens, it just happens all on its own. So if you are living naturally, you'll be able to respond to your natural instincts.

Also, don't be scared off by the naysayers. You came to this for a reason, you started doing this and you feel good. People are going to come at you and say *what about this and what about that*. "Well, what about cholesterol? It's going to cause heart disease! What about red meat? It causes cancer!" Well, what about it? Arm yourself with the facts, know what you're talking about.

Watch my videos, watch Dr. Baker's videos, Dr. Berry's videos. Watch all these and tons of others, Professor Noakes... There are so many people out there that you can learn from - and then you can just dive into the literature.

We all cite our sources, we all talk about different meta-analyses, different studies, that show what we're talking about is for real. That's why we're coming to these conclusions because the evidence really does show this.

I put a lot of links in my videos when I'm talking about specific issues, like cholesterol... and I'll probably put some some links down in the description here, just so you can arm yourself with a few key studies, and go from there!

Also, people get tripped up by thinking that *I have to be perfect.* I personally like living optimally, I like to not have any of this stuff in my system... and that's how I feel the best. And I like feeling my best, so that's what I do.

If you were to slip up, or maybe you were doing this really well for a while and then you had some rice or something else, it's okay! You can start again the next day.

You're going see the contrast now on how good you feel versus how bad you feel when you're eating these things that you don't want. And that's going to reinforce this.

You're going to be like "Wow, I actually do feel so much better! And when I eat just a bit of rice, I actually feel like crap for 4 days, so I really don't want that."

Some people I talk to say that they're doing great, they're feeling amazing. They never felt stronger, never played rugby better. They're just like "I feel great, great, great!"

Then they go to their parents house, like "Well, I had some rice... so I guess, you know, that's it!" No, you can still hang out... I'm not mad at you, just start again. Just start again!

And they kind of look at me "I didn't even think about that." - "Yeah, just go again." We all trip up. You don't have to be perfect right out of the gate. So if something's not exactly perfect to my standards, it's fine! You just keep going, keep working on it. It's not a problem!

A major one that people end up is having problems with, is **alcohol.** Obviously, alcohol is an enjoyable experience. In the social life, it's hard for people sometimes to go out into these alcohol-fueled ventures and social experiences and not drink alcohol.

I'm more used to it because I never drank during the rugby season for many, many years. I did drink a bit but then, after I was 21, I was on antibiotics for a month and I really couldn't drink. So I had to go out sober.

And I was just like "Oh, this is weird, this is strange." Then, the next time, it was... well, it was still weird and strange, but it wasn't as bad. And the third time, it was sort of neutral, I didn't care one way or the other. The fourth weekend, I actually preferred it. I preferred being sober.

I preferred talking to people sober. I thought it was funny when people were drunk. I was able to drive home, I wasn't spending all this money at the bar and I felt great the next day.

I started performing better in rugby, I started performing better at life... and I just thought "Wow, I'm absolutely feeling amazing and I'm playing out of my skin!" - even though I was sick and I had pneumonia.

"I'm going to try this for the rest of season. I'm just going to not drink for the rest of the season." I had the best season of my life! So I'm like "Right, I'm just not going to drink, during the season" after this.

So I'm used to that. You can get used to that, too. But if you do drink alcohol, again: You slip up, you just hop back on. It's not that big a deal! And if you want to drink every now and then and you really don't want to stop that, okay.

That doesn't mean you have to eat pizza, rice cakes and cookies as well. So even if you're just eating meat and drinking water, and then occasionally you're having some drinks - that's still so much better than the other people who are drinking probably more than you are, and are still eating all that other crap. Then as you're going, and you're feeling better and better... and *then* you drink, you're gonna be like "Wow, actually that makes me much worse, that pulls me back!" - for actually a lot longer than you think.

I don't get back to being able to work out to the same level, after I drank, for up to 3 weeks! So that's just not worth it to me. I feel fine, I can do all my daily activities - but when I'm working out to a high level, I definitely don't have the same exercise tolerance or energy level or strength that I do. For seriously full 3 weeks!

So those are some of the main things.

Look: This the easiest diet in the world, it's the easiest way of eating in the world! Keep it that way. You know exactly what you can and can't eat: Meat, water, salt. That's it.

No plants, no sugar nothing artificial. That goes for sauces, seasonings and drinks as well. So what you can eat, you know what you can't eat. There's no confusion here. It is not "Can I have this or that..." - you have hard set rules, you know exactly where you're at.

And if you choose to make exceptions, that's your choice. But you do know what we're trying for here.

You eat as much as you enjoy - not as much as you want, "I want to finish this huge thing!" Well, if your body's telling you to stop and it's not tasting good anymore, when it's becoming a chore to eat - that's when you know you should stop! Your body's telling you that you should stop. So eat as much as you enjoy eating, okay?

Then, eat any time of the day or night, it doesn't matter! Now, I feel better working out, working and doing things on an empty stomach. I've always played hungry, I've always trained hungry. I just feel better that way.

I don't have food in my stomach, my body is trying to digest - and a lot of blood is diverted there, so that I can break this food down. When you go into this rest-and-digest mode, you just feel a bit more chilled out and maybe lethargic.

So for me, I feel a lot better eating towards the end of the day. And I can sleep fine. Some people don't. Some people like to eat earlier, that's fine. It doesn't matter! The only time it really matters is when you're eating carbohydrates.

When you eat carbohydrates late at night, that raises your insulin up – and that blocks growth hormone! Growth hormone gets kicked out, at its highest, about two hours after you go to sleep. It's just part of your natural rhythms.

So when your insulin is up, that's going to block your growth hormone. That's going to actually screw up your body, that's going to screw up your health. Because growth hormone is very important.

So that's when it matters is when you're eating carbohydrates, then you don't want to eat before bed. When you're eating carnivore, eat whenever you like, eat whatever fits your schedule and makes you feel the best.

And then fat: **How much fat** is enough? Well, I like to go by taste, first and foremost. If it tastes good, listen to that.

Also, I like to go by your stools. It's a very easy way to see if you're getting enough fat or not. Your body absorbs fat using bile. It's very hard for your body to absorb fat if you don't have bile. Bile emulsifies the fat and allows your body to absorb it.

Your body can absorb some fat, usually like mid-chain fatty acids, without bile. But to a very small degree. This is just in physiology textbooks, this is just this how this process works.

So most of the fat that you eat - after you run out of bile - will actually just go out in your waste. So you're not going to run into problems eating 'too much fat', because you're not going to absorb it. You're only going to absorb a small percentage of the 'too much fat'.

Unless you're doing something silly, like taking oxbile or something like that, because that's going to force you to absorb more than your body is actually asking for.

So unless you have a problem which requires oxbile, like you don't have a gallbladder anymore and you want to eat a big meal at one time - well, maybe I could see making an exception.

But really, what you should do if you don't have a gallbladder is just eat multiple times during the day to space out those fatty meals. In some people, they make a pseudo gallbladder and that actually works as a normal gallbladder, so they can just eat normally.

If you're not taking oxbile or something like that, you won't absorb more than your body has bile for. Which, I think, means that's more than your body wants. A little bit, but not much. The rest of that goes out.

It's that little bit extra that gets in your stools and it makes them soft. So if you if have hard dry stools and are constipated, that means that you're absorbing every ounce of fat that you're eating - and it's very dry and hard. When you are constipated, that's when it's dry and hard.

You're going to absorb 98 to 99% of the meat that you eat anyway, so you're just going to be going far less often. Don't worry when you're not going more than once every couple of days or once a week. It doesn't matter.

You go when there's waste to get out. If you're eating a whole bunch of non-digestible fiber... it's the same as if you're eating chunks of plastic! You can't digest it, you can't absorb it. It has to go out, so you're just having this stuff come out all the time.

We're just used to this stuff coming out all the time. We think that that's normal - it's not normal, okay? That's your body just trying to get this stuff out of you, because it's not good for you.

If it's dry and hard, that means you need to increase the fat. If it's soft and has a normal consistency, that means you're getting just the right amount of fat. You're getting all the fat that your body wants, from the bile, and a little bit extra.

So you know you've just topped yourself off with the fat. And then, the rest of this goes into the stools and that keeps it soft.

If you eat a lot more then, then that's going to come out quicker. So you're going to get loose stools, that's one of the common causes of loose stools in eating carnivore, is: Way more fat than your body can absorb.

It can also be because people still drink coffee or still use artificial sweeteners, especially sucralose and all the different alcohol sugars. These things cause diarrhea, plain and simple.

A lot of people, they'll get diarrhea when they first start carnivore: "Oh my god, I had these horrible, horrible sh*ts!" - and it's just like "Yeah. Well, are you still drinking coffee? Are you using artificial sweeteners?" Quite often the answer is yes. Coffee will absolutely move things along.

If you are not doing that, if you're only eating meat and drinking water, the likelihood is that you're eating more fat than your body can absorb. Just pull it back, just pull back the fat and you'll be fine.

So I hope that was helpful, just as a little crash course on how to get started - hopefully people can find some use out of that!

Chapter 3

Plants are trying to kill you!

Okay, thank you all for having me here.

The title of my talk is "Plants are trying to kill you!" - which of course is a very provocative title... and is meant to be. But it's trying to make people think about this topic more in depth.

Obviously, this community knows full well about the danger of carbohydrates, how this changes us metabolically, physically and biologically. They can cause a lot of harm.

But we need to remember as well, that there are other chemicals and toxins that exist in the food that we eat, they can also cause harm. Let's think about this.

So just botany 101:

Plants are living organisms and they like to stay living organisms. If you eat them, they die - and so they have defenses, just like any other living organism. While animals can run away or fight back, plants can't - so they use a lot of different things, but poison is one of their main deterrents.

They use these defense chemicals to poison the animals that are trying to eat them. And they have 100s of different ones, geared towards different animals, insects and pathogens, that are trying to eat them.

This is why most plants in the world are inedible. We sort of know this intuitively, if you got lost in the woods here and you ran out of food, you wouldn't be able to eat any random plant. Most of them would make you very sick.

So you have to know exactly what to eat. The reason is because there are these defense chemicals.

Here are just a just a few categories of the ways that plants defend themselves or use.

Lectins is something people are gaining more interest in, there's tons of different kinds of lectins. There's 2500 different plants that use **cyanide,** that we know of.

There's different various

- **Toxins,**
- **Phytates,**
- **Tannins,**
- **Oxalates,**
- **Hormone disruptors,**
- **Nutrient blockers.**
- Things that make you very sensitive to light (**photo sensitivity**) and
- **Nightshades.**

We've known about these for thousands of years and yet, for some reason, we're still eating these things.

So again, just botany, biology 101:
I literally learned this in 7th grade that plants and animals are in an evolutionary arms race: Plants becoming more and more poisonous so less and less animals can eat them, so that they can survive and thrive.

And animals becoming more and more adapted to the specific poisons in specific plants, so that they can eat *that* plant and survive and thrive.

This is where they get their dedicated food resource. It's like koalas and pandas, they eat a very specific diet. If they eat other plants, they will they will get very sick.

The way I came to the way of eating that I do - which is really just meat and water - is 22 years ago, when I was taking cancer biology at the University of Washington in Seattle: We went over how plants use defense chemicals in order to defend themselves.

We were looking at this from a cancer perspective. So we were looking at carcinogens. And we learned, 20 years ago, that brussel sprouts alone had over 136 identified human carcinogens in them.

This is why kids... no one likes brussel sprouts, right? That's why! That bad taste, that bitter taste is your brain and your tongue - which are sophisticated machines - and they can tell you "Hey, this is bad for you, spit it out!"

That's what we would normally, naturally do as a kid. So you give an infant a piece of broccoli, they will hate you for it - you give them a piece of bacon, and their eyes light up.

So we were learning that white cap mushrooms had over 100 known carcinogens But also spinach, kale, lettuce, celery, cabbage, cucumber, broccoli... literally pages and pages of every plant that you ever come across in a grocery store. Not a single one had less than 60 known human carcinogens in them!

They were quite abundant, we have research from Professor Bruce Ames from Berkeley in the 1980s, that actually went into this.

We were quite taken aback by this, obviously. We were very shocked as some of you may be right now. I remember, thinking in my head "Well, but vegetables are still good for you, though. Right?" And our professor must have just read our minds, he like looked at us like *you guys aren't getting this.*

He just said "I don't eat salads. I don't eat vegetables. I don't let my kids eat vegetables. Plants are trying to kill you!" So I was like "Right, forget plants!" and I just stopped.

But: You go to the grocery store and everything has plants, right? Everything either is plants or has plants in the ingredients. And I just walked around and I just came across... it's eggs and meat. I'm like "Okay, so I just eat eggs and meat," and that's what I did for a number of years - and had massive health benefits!

I was playing professional rugby while in University, and my athletic performance, as well as my physical health, just increased dramatically. It was just a night and day difference. And again, still feeling those positive 22 results years later.

So that's the thing, is that most plants will kill most animals. So it's not that some plants are poisonous, some aren't. It's that all plants are poisonous - it's just that certain animals have evolved the ability to defend themselves against specific plants.

But if they eat other plants, they will get sick or even die. So you have pandas and koalas, they eat a very specific diet. It's a very, very monotonous in nature, they don't have this big broad range of things that they eat. They eat very specific things.

There's 340,000 species of plants in the world - koalas eat one. Pandas eat one. Cows, horses, grazing animals eat grasses, and they only eat specific grasses. Then, the leaves the giraffe eats are different from the leaves that a gorilla eats, those are different from the leaves the deer eats, and so on.

And if you mix those leaves around, they all get sick or die.

There is symbiosis between plants and animals, obviously. This is an evolutionary trend in the ecosystem:

You have animals co-evolving with plants. The Great Plains and grasslands have evolved with the big grazing animals. They work together symbiotically.

But also, you can look at fruits, thinking like "Well, fruit... the plant wants you to eat them." Well, maybe - maybe not. They want something to eat them - but not necessarily you! Because certain animals, when they ingest these seeds, those seeds will germinate in their intestine, then that will spawn this plant.

A good example of that is the cassowary bird here in Australia and elsewhere. They eat about 150 different berries and fruits and... those will all kill you!

And they will kill basically any other animal that eats them, because those plants want the cassowary bird to eat them! Because those seeds will not germinate if they don't go through a cassowary bird first. And so, if the Castaway birds leave an area, those plants and trees will die off.

We have this saying „Don't eat the red berries!" This is something that people knew, they identified the red berries. "Don't eat those!" So most fruits are still actually going to be toxic to humans.

This is the study from Professor Bruce Ames from Berkeley.

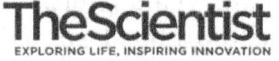

NEWS & OPINION   PUBLICATIONS   CATEGORIES

Home / Archive / July 1989 / Commentary

Man-Made and Natural Carcinogens: Putting The Risks In Perspective

Environmental groups have waged an aggressive campaign to ban Alar, the controversial chemical used on apples to pro- mote uniform ripening and prolong shelf life. They want it banned because a breakdown product of Alar, UDMH, has been shown to cause liver tumors in mice and may pose a cancer risk to humans, especially children. The Alar controversy has heightened people's awareness—and anxiety—about cancer risks of. man-made chemicals in our environment. But little publicit

The Scientist Staff
Jul 9, 1989 / 3 min read

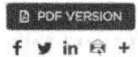

This was published in 1989. He showed that just the natural plants and vegetables contain 10,000 times more naturally

occurring pesticides by weight than the industrial pesticides that we were using on them.

And that they were orders of magnitude times more likely to cause cancer than the industrial pesticides. In this case Alar, which they were looking at specifically, they were trying to actually get it banned.

They were saying "We have to get rid of this, this is poison!" - and it is! But spinach is worse! He had identified, at that point, 42 different toxins that existed in a plethora of different plants. In everything.

I mean, in the article you'll see, it's just every single plant that would exist in the produce aisle. All those vegetables were there and... 42 toxins, 20 of which were shown to be carcinogenic in mice.

Fast forward, 11 years later: When I took cancer biology, we already knew about 136, just in brussel sprouts. So there's probably more now, even more than that.

Even though we've talked about the WHO pushing fake meat and lab meat and all these sorts of things, they still have a page that you can look up that talks about all the natural poisons that are in plants. These "Natural toxins in foods" as they call it.

It does not talk about anything that exists in actual meat, except for the aquatic biotoxins, but this is from algae. The shellfish and fish eat the algae and that can make that toxic. But this is why you avoid things that are infested in that area.

They talk about all sorts of different things like that cyanide, purana cumorins, lectins, solanine, mycotoxins and much more. They talk about poisonous mushrooms as well.

Think about this: We eat mushrooms, but there are over 10,000 varieties of mushrooms in the world. How many of those don't kill you on the spot or give you a religious experience? Right? Yeah, there's like five!

Yet, we think that because these five don't give us an acute stage reaction of that nature - that not only are they safe, but good for you! Which, I think, is a bold assumption to take with your health. The WHO says: *These natural toxins can cause a variety of adverse health effects and pose a serious health threat to both humans and livestock.*

Some of these toxins are extremely potent, these are all things that we eat all the time. They give examples of these things, adverse health effects can be:
- Acute poisoning, ranging from allergic reactions to severe stomach ache, diarrhea, and even death.
- Long-term consequences include effects on the immune- reproductive- or nervous systems... and also cancer.

So speaking about the effects of the mitochondria on cancer: All of those carcinogens in plants damage your mitochondria!

Going into some of the specific categories such as lectins.

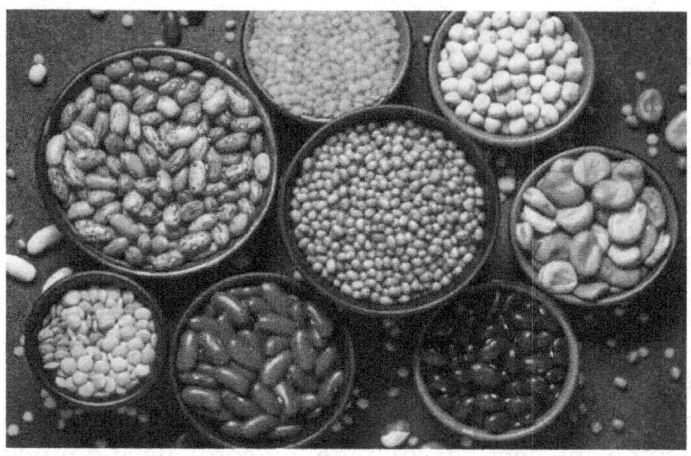

Lectins are proteins that exists in in many, many different plants. They have a bunch of different functions. You actually have lectins in animal meat as well but they don't seem to cause any harm.

These are probably developed anti-pathogenic. They're very, very old and so probably they work against pathogens and insects. But there's obviously a lot of cross-reaction with other forms of life.

These are proteins that can bind to carbohydrates, so they can bind to carbohydrates on the surface of your cells. This is something that's been researched more and more.

Dr. Paul Mason has a really good lecture on just lectins, that he's done at a previous *Low Carb Down Under* event.

And then people like Dr. Paul Saladino... or Dr. Gundry: He wrote an entire book called *The Plant Paradox*, talking about how toxic leptins are ... and then concluded that you should eat a plant-based diet! Which I don't think I would come to that same conclusion.

So we talk a lot about carbohydrates here, how that can affect insulin. How insulin, hyperinsulinemia, can cause all sorts of different problems.

But what we don't necessarily know, is that certain lectins can actually bind to your insulin receptors and bind them more tightly than insulin and cause a greater insulinogenic effect!

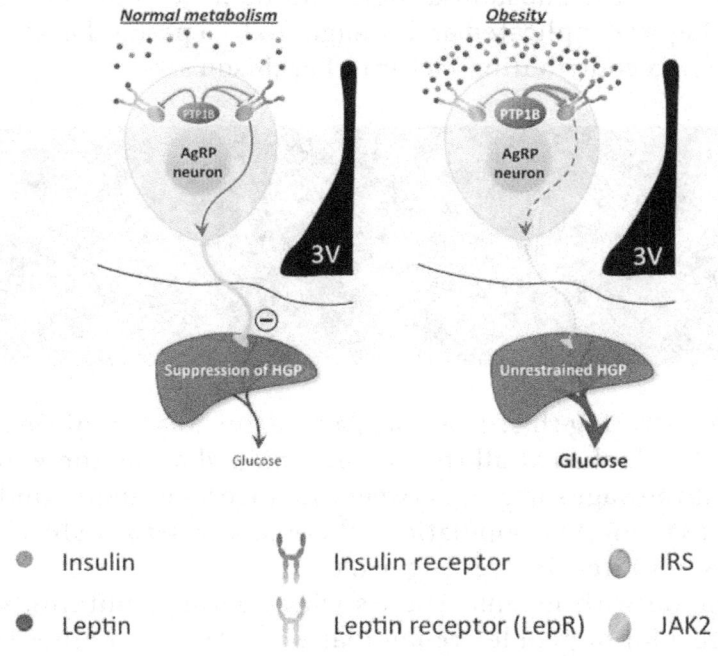

It can also bind to leptin receptors and leptin! Leptin is obviously a satiety signal. It's released from your adipose tissue and your stretch receptors when your stomach is full, it goes to your brain says " We're hungry / We're not hungry, we don't need to eat. We have enough energy."

So you block that, you block that off - which insulin will do as well - then you're not able to see your satiety signals, and you end up overeating. Then you overeat and overeat. This is why we overeat.

This is another reason why people on a ketogenic diet often reduce the amount that they will eat naturally. But sometimes, you'll actually see that the lectins are also having an effect. And when you drop those, people actually lose weight as well.

There was a study, looking at people with an isocaloric intake: One group just removed lectins and they all lost weight - and the other group didn't. They no-lectin group lost a significant amount of weight.

It's also implicated in things like Parkinson's disease: They actually found that lectins can actually track up the vagus nerve and get into the substantia nigra and damage your cells there. Thus, they are implicated and thought to be a part of Parkinson's, or at least a contributing factor to Parkinson's.

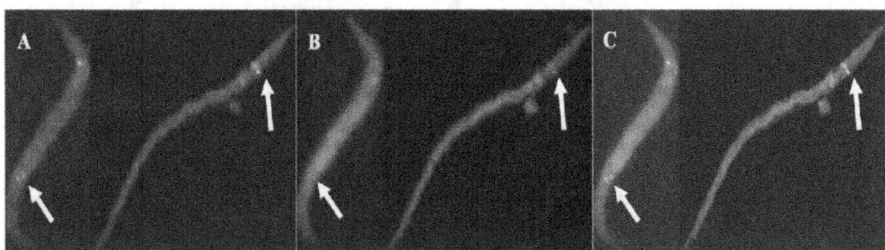

Demonstrating this: There was a study in 2015 out of Denmark where they looked at all the people who had a vagotomy, where they cut the vagus nerve, between the 1970s and 1990 - and they found that in this population, there was a 67% reduction in Parkinson's rates. Interesting, isn't it?

Going on with lectins: There's wheat germ agglutinin, which I'm sure a lot of people are familiar with. This is another lectin, it combines to the carbohydrates surface antigens on your enterocytes, in your intestinal lining.

This can damage them, it can destroy them. It'll also destroy these tight junctions where these cells are literally stuck together, giving barrier protection against things getting in your body that aren't supposed to get in your body.

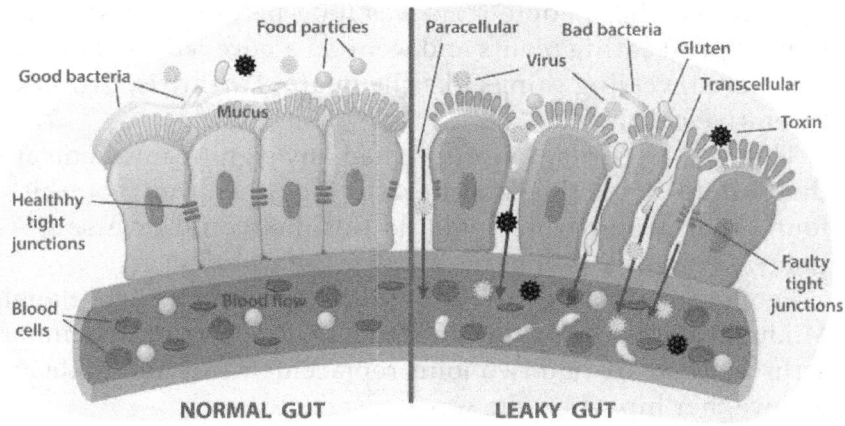

So when you damage those tight junctions, now bacteria and other chemicals that would normally not get into your system - like lectins - will now get into your system and cause all sorts of problems - like bonding to insulin receptors.

Lipopolysaccharides: They are coming from bacteria, they can also bind to Toll-like receptors and this causes an inflammatory cascade.

Within the lectins, there are also chemicals that are capable of molecular mimicry. These are now implicated in autoimmune diseases:

So these lectins obviously are foreign agents, they get into your body and your body doesn't like that, so it attacks them with antibodies. In some people that are genetically susceptible, sometimes they have surface antigens that look similar to these lectins and other foreign objects.

And now, there's a spillover effect of these antibodies - that now attack your normal cells!

This can be demonstrated as far back as the 1800s with Dr. JH Salisbury, after whom the Salisbury Steak was named after.

He did a 30-year research project into optimal nutrition for human beings, and wrote an entire book called *The Relation between Alimentation and Disease*. Basically saying that there is a very strong relationship between disease and what you eat... which is my entire argument. So this has been made way before.

He found that people (this was long before processed sugar) that stopped eating plants and went on a *pure red meat and water diet* were reversing things like rheumatoid arthritis, Crohn's and ulcerative colitis.

This was a century before we had any significant medications that would help, this was devastating when you got this. He found that people who would do this diet could reverse it - and today, people are doing this all over the world.

People may know of Dr. Jordan Peterson, his daughter Mikhaila Peterson, who had such severe juvenile rheumatoid arthritis that she had two joint replacements of her ankle and, I believe, her hip when she was 16 years old!

She went keto first and eliminated out a lot of different toxins - nightshades in particular - and had very good results. Then she even dropped all the salads as well, just went to a pure meat and water diet... now she's off all medications and she's having kids. And: She's healthy!

She has not had a single flare-up. She had salad once - that gave her a flare-up! And she said "Never doing that again!" So that's very interesting as well.

You have these cyanogenic glycosides, these exist in things like cassava root, a very important root which we'll talk about. Also almonds and bitter almonds: They respond to damage.

Once you're chewing an almond, a bitter almond or cassava, that will release this cyanide. So it's normally not in the tissue, just when it's being damaged. This is a defense mechanism.

The cassava root, there's a bitter and there's a sweet. The sweet one, or both of them combined, account for the third most important source of calories in the tropics, and is the primary source of calories for over 500 million people in the world.

So this is a very important source of calories... and it contains cyanide! The bitter cassava will kill you if you eat it, with the amount of cyanide that it has in it - so it has to be specially processed.

They grow the bitter cassava because if they have a problem with herbivores coming around eating their crops... well, they're not going to eat this one, because it'll kill them!

That has to be specially processed, but it doesn't get rid of all the cyanide in it. Long-term exposure to even low-grade cyanide can cause serious thyroid and neurological damage.

We don't have that really as a staple here but people do eat almonds, and people don't realize that 400 to 800 grams of almonds can be a lethal dose of cyanide in an adult. And yet, we give this stuff to kids and sell them in grocery stores, which I think is wild!

Then there's bitter almonds, which are just the inside of like a peach pit or stone, you crack that open. It looks like a little shriveled up almond.

That's very bitter because there's a lot of cyanide in it. And one or two of those - chewed up, crushed up - will release that cyanide, that can be a lethal dose of cyanide in an adult.

There are things that cause direct toxicity: Hemlock is a very well known toxic plant. What it has is a GABBA receptor antagonist, where it will block your GABBA receptor and you'll have intractable seizures and be dead within minutes!

Even half a leaf is enough to kill an adult! Kids that have made little whistles out of the stems in America have been known to be poisoned or even killed. It's very, very toxic.

Oxalates is something that people know a bit about.

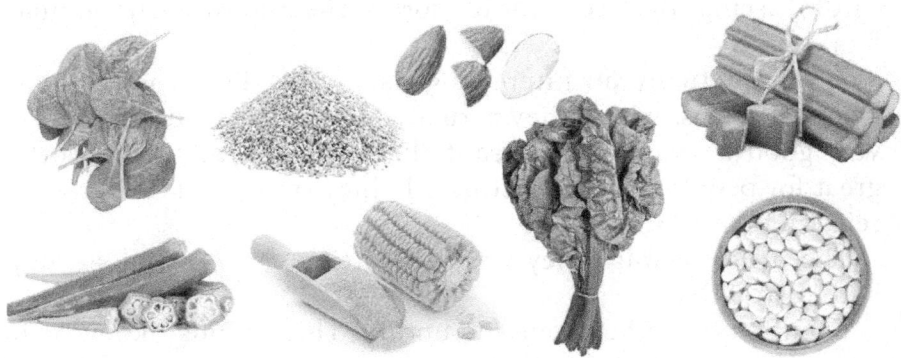

They cause inflammation and damage in your body. They also bind minerals, they are being associated with kidney stones as well.

Tannins: They can block digestive enzymes, slow growth. And, at high enough doses, can even cause kidney damage or liver necrosis.

Seed oils... are just poison!

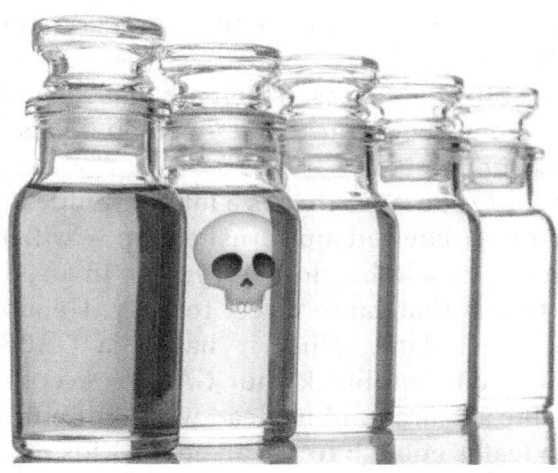

As soon as the oil gets out of the plant, it becomes very unstable and is very pro-inflammatory and oxidative. There's a direct correlation with the rise in seed oils and the rise in cardiovascular disease – but it's sort of the opposite with animal fats.

There's actually an interesting paper that I've read, coming from the 1970s, where they actually found that seed oils were a very good immuno-suppressant. They were saying "This works great for people that are getting a kidney transplant, they're not rejecting their kidneys!"

The problem was: They were all getting cancer! And so they had to stop that.

Then you have hormone disruptors. This sounds like what it is, it disrupts your hormones.

You have phytoestrogens, that can have an estrogenic effect in your body.

I was speaking to someone just last week and they said that their oncologist (because they had breast cancer) didn't want them eating red meat because of all the hormones that were in meat.

But look at this:
- The estrogen that's in red meat for 3 ounces of lean red meat, hormone treated cows, is about 3.9 nanograms of estrogen. Whereas
- The phytoestrogen in soy is over 1,000,000 nanograms per three ounces!

So *Don't eat meat* - what do you replace it with? You replace it with plants that have even more phytoestrogens. The birth control pill has about 35,000 nanograms.

A fertile woman will make over 100,000 nanograms of estrogen a day. So 3.9 nanograms is really not doing anything. So this is taken out of content, and it really matters that it's taken out of that context.

Soy has been shown to reduce reproduction in sheep, it lowers sperm counts and can derange your sex hormone ratios.

Nutrient blockers, these are like the tannins and the oxalates, which can bind different minerals. There are also different things that will just stop your own enzymes from working and digesting your food properly.

Soy and wheat, both have protease inhibitors. These block your protease from your pancreas from actually breaking down normally bioavailable foods, like meat.

The protein that's in plants is not bioavailable. If you think about wheat for example, 80% of the protein in wheat is gluten - and that is completely unavailable to us, to be used as protein.

Then, what little left over is bioavailable and able to be digested, is now going to be hindered by this protease inhibitor. And that wheat protease inhibitor actually also stimulates the toll-like receptor which increases inflammation.

Phytates: You have phytic acid in some plants, these will bind to minerals making mineral salts - and they will stop your body from being able to absorb these, like calcium and magnesium.

Then it's an unbreakable bond! We don't have the machinery to break those two apart. So when we eat these nutrients and we take in things like oxalates and tannins and phytates, we are actually not able to absorb and utilize those nutrients.

Just because it says it on the package, this has this much of this nutrient, doesn't actually mean that that's available and accessible to you. So I think that we really do need to re-examine our recommended daily allowances, our RDAs, because it really does matter whether or not what you're eating is going to change what you actually need, to take in.

Because you're just not going to be absorbing certain things. And all of these RDAs were developed at a time when everyone was eating a mixed diet.

Fiber: There's a lot to do with fiber... but just quickly: It can actually be a physical barrier between the enzymes and your food stuff that's come in and. So it can actually get in the way of that, they won't break down as much.

And then, there's a physical barrier between the breakdown products and the lumen of your intestine. So you won't digest and absorb as many nutrients when you're eating fiber.

This was touted to be a good thing in the 1980s, saying "Oh, you eat more fiber!" This will actually stop you from absorbing nutrients, isn't that great! I don't think that makes any biological evolutionary sense, anyway.

Certainly wouldn't give you a survival advantage, to limit the amount of nutrients you're getting from food. Most animals are starving to death, rather than getting fat in the wild.

Photosensitivity is quite interesting. There's different furanocoumarins that I mentioned before, especially in the citrus and carrot family. Things like lime... just the juice of limes have these furanocoumarins in them.

Then when they get on your skin, they react with light, they are activated by light. And they will bind to proteins and DNA and cause permanent damage. There are cases of kids who have had second-degree burns just from squeezing limes in the sun.

Then you have celery and parsnips: These also have these furanocoumarins which will make you photosensitive.

Celery itself, there's actually an ailment called celery dermatitis, where celery pickers and handlers, that are picking a bunch of celery all the time, they actually get very photosensitive, they get these horrible burns.

These are pictures of a couple of sheep who have gotten into some plants that they normally wouldn't eat. You normally see this in pasture-raised animal livestock, not wild animals... they usually know what to eat.

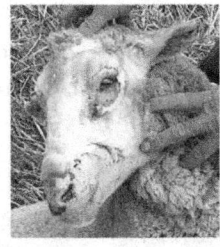 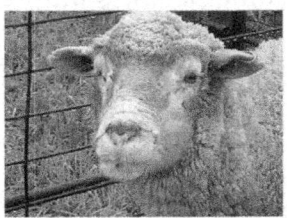

But this is when you're stuck in a passage, you've run out of the things you want to eat – you end up eating things that you wouldn't normally, and you end up getting hurt. This is showing just the burns that these animals can get.

Nightshades: We've known about these things being harmful for thousands of years! Belladonna, tobacco... they create they use a toxin called solanine, among other things.

But we regularly eat potatoes, tomatoes, eggplants, peppers, capsicums - all these things are nightshades. And they all produce solanine. What we forgot when we adopted these things from the new world from, from North and South America, was that:

The people eating them
  a) were poor and didn't really have access to meat, so they sort of had to eat them for survival, and
  b) they processed these things in a very specific way. The tomatoes, when they're green they have a lot more solanine - so you have to wait for them to vine ripen.

Then they would blanch them, take the skin off, take the seeds out. That's where the highest concentration of these poisons were. Potatoes were used to be peeled, now "Oh, well, that's where all the nutrients and vitamins are, in the skin!" That's where all the poison is, too. It's a barrier protection against something going and eating it.

I think most people have grown up with one of their parents telling them that "You have to keep potatoes in a dark cupboard, and if it would turn green, you have to throw it out. It's bad!"

What does that mean? It means it's toxic, it has a toxic level of solanine. Sprout roots too, you have to cut out the entire eye or throw away the whole potato because it's bad.

Apparently, some people's mothers didn't tell them this. So if you look it up: 70 people a year still die from eating potatoes!

This is just a picture of a gate, of a garden in England, that has cultivated and brought together a lot of these very, very toxic plants.

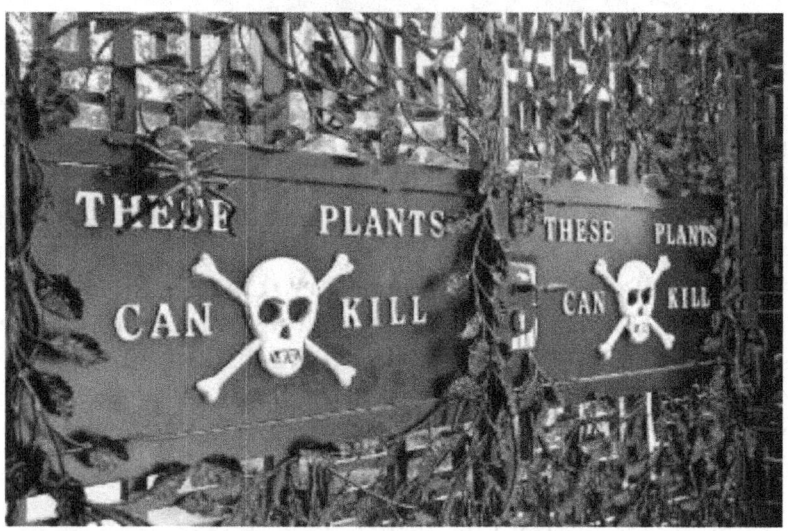

To the extent that: If you get close enough to these things, they can kill you. Just by some of the chemicals that they're exuding. And in fact, the hedge groundskeeper actually succumbed to that and died from one of the plants there!

Just to jump back, think about lectins: Ricin is another lectin. This is a deadly, deadly poison that comes from the skin of castor beans. Even just a few milligrams of this will kill you, invariably.

Coming back to plants as a whole, eating plants:
Do plants contain nutrients?
Yes, plants do contain nutrients, they're living things. They have things that are good for other living things.

But this comes at a price - and they're also not as bioavailable as we think. This is why we need to redo these RDAs, because it's a very different story if you are excluding these nutrient blockers and digestive disruptors.

So the RDAs for someone doing keto or just meat, is going to be very different than otherwise.

Does it have anything vital, essential? Nutrients that you have to have, that you cannot get from meat?

Well, no. It doesn't. And we have endless examples of this, going back through antiquity.

But even current examples today, the Masai, the Inuit... and all of our ancestors have lived through previous ice ages, where we didn't have access to all these different sorts of plants - and they really relied on a meat-based diet. They did fine!

I'm fine and I've been doing this for literally decades... and there are other people that have been doing it for longer than I have, coming from a Western European background.

Does it cause harm?

Yes, I think I think that it does. I hope that I've made that point clear to you.

Plants are not part of an optimal human diet...

Contain nutrients?	✓
Any vital nutrients not found in meat?	✗
Cause harm?	✓

The Toxin Theory of Modern Disease
Plants have toxins they use in self defense. Humans today are not suffering from chronic illnesses, but from poisoning and lack of species appropriate nutrition

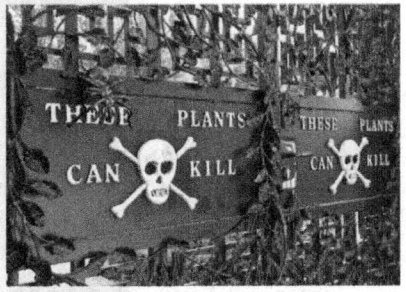

I mean, there's thousands and thousands of different defense chemicals that these things use, and I have just sort of scratched the surface of these things. But: They do!

Now, why is this important to us as people, and specifically doctors?

Well, the fact is these defense chemicals cause a large burden of harm and illness in the population - and we're not treating it as such! We're thinking "Oh, this is a disease. We need to treat the disease."

We're not recognizing: *This is a toxicity - we need to remove the toxin!* Okay? And let the body heal naturally.

We're pacing over this, saying "Well, here's all these treatments..." not thinking what the root cause is.

I'm pretty sure no one here would argue that type 2 diabetes is caused by a *Metformin deficiency*. Right? So we need to look at what's causing this. I think that it's these toxins!

78

In animal husbandry, we actually have known about this for a long time: There are a number of different ailments that are directly attributed to the animal eating the wrong thing.

Such as the

- Blind staggers
- Slobbers
- Paralytic tongue
- Big head
- Limp neck
- Crazy Cow syndrome

...and we recognize these as coming from eating the wrong thing.

I think, now as doctors, we need to recognize that a lot of our chronic diseases are actually plant toxicities. And what I would argue, is that the so-called *chronic diseases* that we treat are not diseases per se, but toxicities and malnutrition.

Toxic buildup of a species inappropriate diet and a lack of species-specific nutrition. Namely: Too many plants, not enough meat.

So that's what I call just the
Toxin Theory of Modern Disease.

I think we're looking at this incorrectly. And because we're looking at this incorrectly, we're going to get incorrect treatments.

Just like, you get the wrong diagnosis in the hospital, you start someone on the wrong treatment, that's not going to help them. It's going to hurt them.

I think that's what we're doing - and that's why we're not having very good results, even though we've spent billions trying to treat these diseases.

They're only getting worse.

That because we're looking at them incorrectly. So as every doctor's been saying the last years: "Make sure you eat your vegetables"... obviously *don't!* Don't eat your veggies!

At least something to think about, anyway.

Thank you very much!

References

Natural pesticides in vegetables. Bruce Ames
http://www.garfield.library.upenn.edu/papers/vethumtoxicology31(6)p589y1989.html

Bruce Ames' article to *The Scientist*
https://www.thescientist.com/?articles.view/articleNo/10489/title/Man-Made-and-Natural-Carcinogens--Putting-The-Risks-In-Perspective/ Science
(244:755-7, May 19,1989)

WHO Natural Plant Toxins https://www.who.int/news-room/factsheets/detail/natural-toxins-in-food?fbclid=lwAR2j8SyhGBJzPL1lro51J-4BLNRKKVYGAN344Um9ACLAc-Q13jckUYSe7DY

Polyunsaturated fats are immunosuppressants
http://www.functionalps.com/blog/2011/09/22/polyunsaturated-fatssuppress-the-immune- system/?fbclid=lwAROrt89m|WAx8BO2FgK3FW7L6nFgwjS6|PvnblrBRKIE-y4NJ2Dg0xojNg

Hormones in food
https://newsroom.unl.edu/announce/beef/2846/15997

Leaky gut https://jamesclinic.com/how-leaky-gut-affects-autoimmunediseases

Lectin binds to leptin
https://www.sovereignlaboratories.com/blog/lectin-vs-leptin-makesdifferent/

Molecular mimicry https://www.moleculeralabs.com/education-series-2017-molecular-mimicry-autoimmune-disease/

Elemental diet found to be as or more effective as prednisone for acute Crohns exacerbations in clinical trial:
https://www.bmj.com/content/288/6434/1859.abstract

Elemental diet better than steroids in children; clinical trial https://adc.bmj.com/content/62/2/123.short

Elemental diet better than polymeric diet in treating Crohn's and keeping in remission. Quick absorption, less stress on cut, EG fiber opposite of this.

https://www.sciencedirect.com/science/article/pii/014067369090936Y

Exclusion diet keeps Crohn's patients in remission for up to 51 months, or current rate less than 10% per annum, contrasted with starch-based high fiber diet keeping zero patients in remission; clinical trial
https://www.sciencedirect.com/science/article/pii/S0140673685914977

Fasting mimicking diet shows benefit in inflammatory bowel disease, promotes GI regeneration and reduces IBD pathology in clinical trials
https://www.sciencedirect.com/science/article/pii/S2211124719301810

Fasting mimicking diet as treatment protocol for IBD
https://scholar.google.com.au/scholar?hl=en&as_sdt=0%2C5&q=fasting+mimicking+diet+as+treatment+for+IBD&btnG=#d=gs_qabs&t=1653632919273&u=%23p%3DHlwZjz_TjwcJ

Vagotomy & Parkinson's' Disease
https://scholar.google.com/scholar?hl=en&as_sdt=0%2C5&q=vagotomy+reduced+risk+for+Parkinson%27s&btnG=#d=gs_qabs&t=1665465081656&u=%23p%3DAbXUef7BQYKJ

Vagus nerve tracking
https://www.frontiersin.org/articles/10.3389/fnut.2016.00007/full

Maternal fibre associated with T1D in offspring
https://www.ncbi.nlm.nih.gov/pmc/articles/PMC6283375/

Chapter 4
The hard facts about cancer and diet. With Professor Thomas Seyfried

Hello everyone! Today's interview will be with Professor Thomas Seyfried, in what I think is probably the most important interview I've ever done.

Professor Seyfried is one of the world's foremost experts in cancer, cancer biology and research. He has actually shown, quite conclusively, that our understanding of cancer is all wrong.

And by being all wrong, our approaches to treating it are all wrong - and so we're not getting the results that we should and could be. So please, if you are a cancer patient or you know anyone with cancer, tell him or her about the information provided in the following conversation.

Dr. Chaffee:
I'm here today with a very special guest, someone whose work I've long admired: Professor Thomas Seyfried of Boston College. Professor Seyfried, thank you so much for joining us! How are you?

Prof. Seyfried:
Thank you very much Anthony, it's a real pleasure to be here! I'm fine.

Dr. Chaffee:
Thanks! For people that aren't familiar with your work, can you tell us a bit about yourself? What you do and some of your current projects.

Prof. Seyfried:
Well, I'm a Professor of biology at Boston College. I teach cancer metabolism, every semester, to a select group of undergraduate and graduate students.

I also teach general biology to the folks that are not science majors. Like the economists, the political science folks and the English majors. To try to increase scientific literacy among the population.

We have a very active research program, supported by private foundations. Our goal is to develop diet / drug therapies for managing cancer. All types of cancer.

So that's our big thrust right now: What are the most efficacious diet / drug combinations that can manage cancer, without inducing toxicity to any of the normal cells or tissues of our body. What we do then, is:

We collaborate with clinics that are treating cancer patients throughout the world. And we share the knowledge that we have from our pre-clinical studies with the directors of these clinics, so that they can start applying metabolic therapy - non-toxic metabolic therapy - to their patients in these clinics.

And the success that we're hearing coming back is quite astonishing! This is working!

We ferret out everything before we put it on patients, and my clinical colleagues will then apply it to the patient. So we have everything planned in advance and we get forward-feedback information.

What we do is:

We tweak our systems in-house here, to see if we can improve therapeutic efficacy, and then share that again with the clinical groups. And we're constantly making more and more advances and perfections in the strategy - that will eventually become the standard of care for all cancer patients.

That is: **Metabolic therapy.**

Dr. Chaffee:
I certainly hope so! I've read some of your papers, specifically on glioblastoma multiforme. I'm in neurosurgical residency at the moment, so that's obviously the most common thing that we see. It's an absolutely devastating disease.

Obviously, without any sort of treatment, on average people live about 3 months. With treatment, they make it 15 to 18 months. This is a very devastating illness to watch someone have to go through.

You obviously have copious amounts of publications... some of your publications talk about cancer as a metabolic disease. Specifically, as a dysfunction of the mitochondria. Can you talk a bit about that?

Prof. Seyfried:

Yes, this goes back to the work of Otto Warburg in the 1920s, 30s and 40s, where he defined that cancer originated from damage to mitochondria - and that then elicits a whole series of changes: Forcing the cell into a fermentation mechanism to survive.

We have validated and confirmed Warburg's original finding. In order to do that, I went through the scientific literature, looking at electron micrographs, high magnification of mitochondria and tissues...

Because you can't see them under light microscopy. In order to look at the structure of the mitochondria in the cytoplasm of the cell, you really need electron microscopy.

And I looked at all the major cancers, probably representing 95% of all cancer deaths are caused by these kinds of cancers. I went back through the 1950s, 60s, 70s...

Because back then, in a lot of medical schools, people would be looking at cancer tissue with electron microscopy. Then you go to those papers and you look what they found with respect to the number and structure of the mitochondria in those cancer tissues - and invariably, they were abnormal, structurally.

Even if one were to isolate them and look at the biochemistry, it was abnormal. *So we have never found normal mitochondria in any kind of a major cancer!*

If you don't have normal mitochondria, that means your cells are not going to be able to generate energy through normal respiratory systems, like oxidative phosphorylation [Ox-Phos].

And this is exactly what Warburg said! He said mitochondria, oxidative phosphorylation, becomes irreversibly damaged in all cancers, regardless of where they come from. Thereby forcing them into a fermentation mechanism. And that's what the characteristics of all cancer cells are: They ferment!

Warburg knew glucose was... the lactic acid fermentation, derived from glucose, was the major fuel at that time. We have now defined glutamine as a second fermentable fuel.

The field thought for many years that glutamine was being respired. No, it's not respired, it's fermented. So the two fermentation pathways that drive the majority of cancers are a sugar fermentation and an amino acid fermentation. Without the glucose and glutamine, no cancer cell can survive!

So our goal is to scientifically validate this fermentation mechanism for glutamine and show how Warburg was right in his original description - but he also did not have new information which would clarify and resolve this entire cancer issue back then.

And we're in the process of doing this right now.

Dr. Chaffee:

Yeah, that's fantastic! So what are some of the things that can disrupt the mitochondria, to make them precipitate cancer. How does that go about?

How does this actually precipitate the genetic mutations, that we see and attribute blame to as causative - but you're saying that that's actually a knock-on effect.

Prof. Seyfried:

Yeah, the mutations are all downstream epiphenomena. As are most symptoms of what people are studying today, they are all downstream:

The angiogenesis, the failure in apoptosis, all these kinds of things. They're all downstream of the original damage to the mitochondria.

So to answer specifically your question: It's called the oncogenic paradox. And this paradox has perplexed the cancer field for decades!

In other words: How is it possible that you could get cancer from a whole range of different kind of insults? What is the common pathophysiological mechanism that could underlie this range of cancer initiators?

For example, some women may get breast cancer from a clogged milk duct, another one may get it from some sort of viral infection. Another one may get it from a unhealed wound.

There's a whole variety of different ways that could elicit breast cancer.

You can consider the same thing for colon cancers, bladder cancers, lung cancers or any other kind of cancers.

Of course, smoking would damage the mitochondria in lung tissues and possibly other tissues.

- Intermittent hypoxia
- Radiation
- Chronic inflammation

Any of these kinds of insults could *damage the mitochondria* of a cell in a particular tissue, leading to dysregulated cell growth in that tissue.

And the definition of cancer is cell division out of control, or dysregulated cell growth. How does that happen?

It happens from damage to the mitochondria in populations of cells, in a particular tissue - eliciting a dysregulated growth. And that's the oncogenic paradox.

So you don't always get cancer from a single insult, it could come from a variety of insults. The bottom line is that you end up with cells that are dysregulated in their cell growth - all of which are fermenting.

And it's important to recognize that the mitochondrion of our cells is the controller of the cell cycle! So when that organelle becomes defective, the cell falls back into a dysregulated cycle.

This is the way all cells on the planet evolved before oxygen came into the atmosphere, 2.5 billion years ago. We had living cells on the planet before oxygen was in the atmosphere. And: They were all fermenting and they all had dysregulated cell growth.

So the cancer cells are simply falling back on these ancient pathways that have always existed, even before respiration... even before the origination of the mitochondria! So the cells are just simply falling back.

And as long as they have fermentable fuels in the environment, they're very difficult to kill. Radiation and chemo and all these things that we use, are not at the heart of the problem.

As a matter of fact, some of the standards of care actually facilitate the availability of fermentable fuels, making the management of the disease impossible!

That's why the current standard of care makes no sense, when one considers the origin of the disease in the concepts of evolutionary biology.

Dr. Chaffee:
I did read a study a number of years ago, where it spoke about people going on a ketogenic diet. Speaking specifically about using ketosis, about mitochondria specifically.

Showing that when in a state of ketosis, your mitochondria were more efficient - and they also increased in number! Is this some sort of mechanism that would protect from cancer?

What is it about eating carbohydrates and not being in ketosis, that just jams up our mitochondria so much?

Prof. Seyfried:
Well, I don't think the carbohydrates jam up the mitochondria. What happens is that excessive amounts of carbohydrates cause an inflammatory condition in the body.

And it's this elevated inflammation, the state of an inflammation, that contributes to the damage.

Sugar itself is not a carcinogen. However: Chronic excessive consumption of carbohydrates can put the body in an imbalanced nutritional state - and that's what elicits the disease.

It's not only cancer, it's
- Type 2 diabetes
- Alzheimer's disease
- Cardiovascular disease

It's essentially: All of the major chronic diseases that we are currently suffering from are the result of excessive amounts of carbohydrates in the diet.

We as a species did not evolve to eat large amounts of carbohydrates. It was only a seasonal kind of situation. A ripe fruit, a ripe berry or something like this would be so sweet. Maybe honey.

It wasn't chronic exposure to high levels of carbohydrates, that are coming from the foods that we presently have in our societies. And that is ultimately the origin of the majority of chronic diseases that we have:

A diet that is does not fit our evolutionary past.

Dr. Chaffee:
Yeah, I would 100% agree with you on that. And that's something that I've argued for a while now.

Which is that the chronic diseases that we're treating nowadays - exactly as you've outlined - are not diseases per se, but toxicities and malnutrition. A toxic buildup of a species inappropriate diet and a lack of species specific nutrition.

Prof. Seyfried:
Yeah.

Dr. Chaffee:
You build up these toxins, as I mentioned to you before this interview.

I got into this when I took cancer biology, we talked about carcinogens at the time, this was 20 years ago... and we were told that there's 136 known carcinogens just in brussel sprouts, and over 100 in mushrooms, and so on.

So plants are obviously using defense chemicals to stop predation or deter predation. These can build up and cause toxic effects on our body.

Prof. Seyfried:
Well, I think that's true for the industrially produced vegetables. I think organic vegetables, using appropriate natural fertilizers, are safe to eat.

The problem is that organic foods are hard to come by. It's not known whether they're really organic or not. I don't think there's any regulatory commission of free-range animals or organic plants.

I mean, this is what we evolved to eat: They were all organic, 50,000 years ago. There was no industrial harvesting of foods.

But I think that organically grown vegetables, with natural fertilizers, I think those would be very healthy. Along with any other free range meat products or things like this.

The problem is: They're not convenient for the majority of people in the society. Driving up to McDonald's, getting a hamburger is a hell of a lot easier than going out and shooting a deer in the woods!

Dr. Chaffee:
Yeah.

Prof. Seyfried:
You know, it's just the way our society is. Our demands on our time and what we do prevent us from actually rebalancing our physiology. But yet, we put ourselves at risk for cancer and all these other chronic diseases by the convenience of our lifestyle.

Dr. Chaffee:
I certainly agree that with any sort of a whole foods approach, you're going to be in much better stead.

One of the things that I wanted to mention is this data from a guy from Berkeley, Professor Bruce Ames. He published in 1989 some work, looking at an comparison of *Alar*, which was a pesticide used on apples at the time... they were trying to ban it.

He actually showed - looking specifically in mushrooms - that mushrooms had around 10,000 times the amount of natural insecticides and pesticides by weight as the Alar would get sprayed on these plants. And that this amount of plant carcinogens was thus way more likely to cause cancer than the pesticide ones.

But to your point: I agree 100%, obviously pesticides and insecticides, these are toxic by design. They're trying to kill insects from eating them. So certainly, that's going to make things a lot worse.

Prof. Seyfried:
Well, in my book I showed that a lot of these so carcinogens that you just mentioned *[He is talking about the Alar carcinogens]*, they're taken up in mammalian cells and they actually cause the mitochondria to fluoresce. Biofluorescence.

So those carcinogens are going right to the mitochondria, damaging the mitochondria. Which is then the first step...

The first step in the initiation of cancer is to disrupt oxidative phosphorylation, OxPhos. And only cells that can upregulate a fermentation mechanism as the result of this damage, only those cells can become cancer cells!

Cells that can not upregulate fermentation rarely if ever become tumorigenic. Cells of cardiomyocytes, they can't switch from OxPhos to fermentation. Neurons in the brain rarely become tumorigenic. It's the glial cells, not the neuron. Neurons can't ferment for very long.

So only cells that have the capacity to replace respiration with fermentation can become cancer cells.

Dr. Chaffee:
That's very interesting! And I think that's a good illustration of what the actual mechanism is.

Prof. Seyfried:
Yeah. I mean, it becomes very clear once you understand the biology of the problem. Understanding how we get it and, and more importantly, understanding how we manage it. That becomes very logical.

The problem is: This information is not known by the majority of oncologists or scientists in the field.

Dr. Chaffee:
Absolutely. In addition to that, with my sort of endeavors into nutrition and how this affects disease: Even just the idea that diabetes and heart disease are caused by eating a lot of carbohydrates and sugar, a lot of people really don't know it.

Doctors don't know about these things, nutritionists as well. They still are on the same "Cholesterol will kill you-" idea. Which I think has been thoroughly debunked.

Prof. Seyfried:
Well, it's been debunked - but everybody's popping the statin tablets! Obviously, they still think cholesterol has a big role in cardiovascular disease. Triglycerides.

You're absolutely right. And in the cancer wards, they still give the cancer patients sugar, coke and ice cream, cake... and they say glucose has nothing to do with cancer.

There's such a lack of knowledge, it's profound, it's unbelievable! The lack of knowledge on the part of the healthcare industry, as to what should and should not be done to keep people healthy.

Dr. Chaffee:
Yeah that's one of the things, I was a bit upset there...

Because I see this every day in the hospital. You know, I see the food that they feed them. It's just sugary carbs, that's it. There's almost no meat, there's certainly no fat. There's a bit of dairy... but it's always like chocolate milk, as opposed to just normal milk. Just garbage.

I'm going around seeing our brain tumor patients who just underwent surgery... and here they are, eating all this sugary nonsense.

And I just can't help but think "This is what gave you this problem in the first place - and we're just shoveling it into your face!"

Prof. Seyfried:
Yeah, it drives the tumor. What we also found:

I published a major paper on this, with the standard of care for brain cancer: The very treatments that are used, the radiation, as well as Temazolamide, they free up massive amounts of glucose and glutamine in the tumor micro environment - making long-term survival very, very rare!

So it's the therapies themselves that... In other words, it's bad enough to have a glioblastoma - it's even worse to use standard of care to treat it! Because you've more or less signed and sealed the death certificate of this patient.

The human brain should rarely - if ever - be irradiated. This is nonsense, this has to stop!

I published a clear paper on how the radiation breaks apart the glutamine- glutamate cycle in the brain, freeing up massive amounts of glutamine. And the steroids they give these patients increase blood sugar.

So the two fuels necessary causing cancer cells to grow out of control are made available, in abundant quantities, by the very treatments that we're doing to these patients.

Dr. Chaffee:
Yeah...

Prof. Seyfried:
We have made no advance in glioblastoma therapy in almost 100 years. My most recent paper shows, in 100 years...

We have a telescope that now orbits 1 million miles from earth to look at the very origins of our solar system - we do that, and yet we've made no advance in glioblastoma!

And many other cancers. Once you have metastatic lung cancer, a colon cancer, the survival is so much less. Because the treatments we're using contribute to the demise of these patients. It's unbelievable!

Dr. Chaffee:
Yeah, absolutely.
Prof. Seyfried:
A tragedy, it's actually a tragedy.
Dr. Chaffee:
Right, and chemo can be so hard on people.

I don't know what people are more concerned with: Like getting cancer - or getting cancer and realizing that means they need chemo. Because I've had friends, and obviously patients, devastated by these treatments.
Prof. Seyfried:
Yeah, I think they fear the treatment as much as they do the disease. They think their hair is going to fall out, they're going to bleed from the gums, they're going to be sick and tired all the time. Some people recover really well.

Actually, there are some reports now that show water-only therapeutic fasting can significantly reduce some of the toxic effects of chemotherapy.

But my point is: Why would you want to use chemotherapy, when we know we just have to pull the plug on the fermentable fuels? With diet and drugs that aren't so toxic? Especially when under therapeutic ketosis.

I mean, there's a clear framework and strategy for managing cancer without toxicity. The biggest problem is there is no business model to support this. Which is the singular greatest inhibitor of moving this forward.

People haven't found out how to make money on metabolic therapy. Yet! That's the biggest problem. It's not the patient that should be benefited, it's how to make revenue from this.

I think the entrepreneur will come, and the entrepreneur will figure out how to do this. I'm not that kind of a person. My job is: *How do we keep cancer patients alive with a higher quality of life, beyond what they were ever predicted to have.*
Dr. Chaffee:
Yeah. I suppose a good business model would be just setting up clinics, that have this treatment regime and actually get results - and then people will go to them.
Prof. Seyfried:
We're doing that now, actually. We have some clinics...

But some of the drugs that we use like a 6-Diazo-5-oxo-Lnorleucine (DON) is not available to the public. And it really bothers me, because that was used on children and cancer patients and patients with other indications in the past.

But yet, if you try to get it, the drug administration would say "It's not for human use, not for human consumption." That should not be, because that drug is very powerful, especially when used in ketosis.

We did the experiments. We showed the results... and hundreds and hundreds of cancer patients are emailing me "How do I get this drug?"

The answer is "Write your senator or congressman! They should make this legal to get!" Because it's a drug that has to be repurposed.

It was used on cancer, but it wasn't used in the right way. If you don't know how to use the tool, it's not going to give you the outcome that you would expect.

They say "Oh, it's too toxic" - relative to what? Chemo and radiation? No, not even close!

So we have a drug available right now, that can be used to reduce cancer in so many patients - when used with nutritional therapeutic ketosis. We've already shown how it works, and it works really well. And it should be used right now! But it's not, because there's no profit in this drug.

So when there's no profit, we can't use it, regardless of the patient. Can you believe this is? This is what we call a moral issue.

Dr. Chaffee:
Is there any way to sort of push through, getting it approved by the FDA? To get this going? Or is it there's just no money...

Prof. Seyfried:
You know, I think it's all revenue generation. I'm sorry to say that. The FDA will approve drugs *if there's a proof of concept*. Nothing could be stronger than the proof of concept of how this drug DON works with ketosis. Nothing is as strong as this!

Yet, it won't be approved - because there's no revenue to be generated from this.

It's a business model! People have to realize that is a revenue generating disease. Hospitals use drugs and radiation because they generate so much revenue from the insurance companies.

So are we interested in keeping people alive longer? Yes! But it seems only, if it can be associated with revenue generation.

If it's not associated with revenue generation, I'm sorry: We have to sacrifice those cancer patients. There it is.

Dr. Chaffee:

Yeah. I'm in Australia at the moment, so a there's a public and a private health care system here. But regarding the public system: Obviously, this is coming from the government. And there are massive delays within this system, so it can actually take 4.5 years for someone to get into our clinic.

With like radiculopathy, a compressed nerve in their spine, that needs surgery. 4 and a half years is our current wait list for that. So there are a lot of delays and there are a lot of issues.

But we deal with a lot of cancer as well, those get obviously treated right away because it's a life or death emergency. But the government really tries hard to not pay for anything that gets done, and they put a lot of roadblocks in the way.

And I just wonder: Wouldn't this be something that would be attractive to them? Because this is eminently more cheaper than the actual standard treatments. I think that... Well, you may have some ideas?

Maybe it's that a lot of hospitals and systems around the world that have a public model, generally try to emulate the guidelines set in America in the private system with the insurance, sort of driving things.

Prof. Seyfried:

Yeah, you would think so. You would think this would be the best thing for governments to cut their medical bills. No. No, no. There's a force, there's a power that's controlling this. Even though the governments would like to do it.

The IRB, institutional review boards, have shut down this so many times. They want to do standard of care first, before they do metabolic therapy. Why?

Well, there's something else going on here. And again, it has to do with the control of the entire medical system. What we call standard of care.

Care standard of care should have never been written in granite. But it seems to have been written in granite.

In other words: You can use metabolic therapy only after you demonstrate that conventional chemo and radiation don't work. Now, for glioblastoma, 99% of the time they don't work!

So why do we have to continue to push ineffective therapies? And once we realize they don't work, then we maybe want to do metabolic therapy?

No, no, no. You should do metabolic therapy first! That's the number one. Do metabolic therapy first, and then you'll be shocked at how you won't need toxic radiation and chemicals.

And that is not what the system wants to hear. Period.

Dr. Chaffee:
Well, that obviously needs to change somehow. I don't know...

Prof. Seyfried:
Yes, but who's going to change it?

Dr. Chaffee:
Right, I don't know.

Prof. Seyfried:
The bottom line is:

You just keep treating patients with metabolic therapy and let the patients be the advocates of what's going on. Let them go out and tell people what they did. "Why are you still alive? How come you're not dead? You should have been dead three years ago, and you're out here working in your garden!"

He'll tell you. Those guys will be more than happy to tell you what they did.

Dr. Chaffee:
Well, that's the thing... not even to the extent that you're talking about, actual treatment modalities with diet and drugs.

I had a friend of mine who was diagnosed with glioblastoma multiforme, about 6 years ago. And I had already been involved in this sort of research, seeing a lot work from yourself and others.

I just said "Hey look, there's a lot of evidence here that suggests that at least being on a ketogenic diet is going to be very beneficial" - I sort of pitched a carnivore diet because that's my thing.

But she didn't do a whole carnivore diet, diet she did more keto. But she had a lot more meat. She cut out the carbs, she stopped drinking... and she's now 6 years still alive! At 5 years, she had an MRI - and she had no sign of disease!

Unfortunately, it did come back in her sixth year. So she's sort of undergoing a further debulking. But 5 years and her 5-year MRI was clear. That's almost unheard of with GBM.

Prof. Seyfried:
Well, see: Those kinds of cases need to need to be written up. The patient that we wrote up, Pablo Kelly, who has a website and talks about his survival:

He chose no standard of care, just metabolic therapy. And he was on a carnivore kind of diet.

So he's out now 8 years. And his tumor is not gone, it's there. He has a debulking surgery every three years. No radiation or chemo.

I'll give you the full story, a very kind of a colorful guy from Devon, England. He used the carnivore procedure. No carbs, he cut all that stuff out. And he's still going fine, he's had two children.

He was 26 when he was diagnosed, lived a 'horrible lifestyle', as he said. Alcohol, drugs and bad food, all that kind of stuff. Of course, after his tumor diagnosis, he became very pristine in what he was doing - and he's still doing fine!

There's two things we think need to happen.
1) Avoiding the standard of care
2) Switching your entire diet lifestyle over to zero or very low carbohydrate

Whether you do that with carnivore or whether you do it with plants... you can you can do it with either or.

We developed the *glucose-ketone index calculator (GKI)*, to allow people to know whether or not they're in a state of nutritional ketosis by blood markers. You can do Keto-Mojo, that's a blood glucose-ketone meter.

So the cancer patient knows what is going on metabolically.

And when Pablo went off his diet a little bit, the tumor started to grow again - and you could see it on MRI! And immediately, he threw himself back into a very low GKI index. Then, you could see the tumor stopped growing. It was very clear.

Cancer cells can't burn ketones or fats, they only can burn glucose and glutamine. But there's no diet that will target glutamine.

So patients always ask "Oh, what am I going to eat to target glutamine?" Glutamine is the most abundant amino acid in our body, it's not gonna work with any kind of diet I'm afraid.

Now, I'm shocked at how long people can live with just ketogenic diets or these kinds of things. But if we ever married those diets with the glutamine targeting drug DON, I think we could eliminate these tumors in the majority of people very quickly!

We're not doing that. We're not doing the very things we need to do to make cancer a very manageable disease, without suffering great toxicity.

Why are we not doing this? Because
- Nobody knows about it, they simply don't know it. And
- The ones that are in charge don't want to believe it

If you go to most of the oncology centers, they say "There's no evidence to support metabolic therapy. If it were so important and effective, we would all know about it"

Wrong! You wouldn't know about it. You're dealing with huge profits for an entire industry here, let's be honest. Right?

Dr. Chaffee:

Absolutely, yeah. So with the DON, going to the drug and diet cocktail: Obviously, they're not letting us use this in humans. But you've done quite extensive animal models and experiments, is that right?

Prof. Seyfried:

Yes. We've looked at it in a variety of metastatic and invasive brain cancers and things like this. I mean, all of these drugs... DON was used in humans! It was used in little kids with leukemia.

So it's not like it's a drug that's never been used in humans. Of course it's been used. It's in malaria treatments, there's a lot of ways that that drug has already been used. But not for cancer.

Of course, don't you think the pharmaceutical industry knows about glutamine targeting? Sure they do!

So what they do is: They build drugs that are not nearly as effective as DON, patent that drug and then throw that drug out on the cancer population, but never using keto with it.

You get some therapeutic benefit, maybe. But you're not going to get the full therapeutic benefit.

Cancer can be managed with drug / diet cocktails. People need to know that!

We clearly showed how nutritional ketosis can facilitate the delivery of these drugs to tumor cells, three times more. That means you can lower the doses, reduce the toxicity and increase the efficacy of the whole process.

We know the framework, we know how to manage cancer. Without toxicity. The problem is: It won't be used in the clinics - for a variety of different reasons.

The people themselves have to rise up and say "I want metabolic therapy! „Forget about all this crazy nuking and poisoning people. I mean, it's not based on we understand the biology of the disease to be.

So who's going to make the change? The guys at the top medical schools? No. It's going to be the people themselves.

Who will benefit most from metabolic therapy? The cancer patients will benefit most from metabolic therapy. They need to understand this, they need to rally, they need to do something. Put pressure on your government officials and these kinds of things. Then it will happen.

It's never going to happen when you're trying to convince Big Pharmacy and big medical schools that metabolic therapy is the way to go. Because it's not going to generate the replacement revenue. So you have to have something that's going to give replacement revenue.

In my mind, I want to see how many people can survive long term. Like your friend, like Pablo Kelly. Like many others who should have been dead a long time ago. People who are living a hell of a lot longer with a higher quality of life.

What's wrong with that? Why is this being resistant? Why is there resistance against this? Makes no sense to me.

Dr. Chaffee:
Yeah, especially with something like cancer. If there was ever something to rally behind, I think cancer is it. Anyone you talk to around the world, they always have sympathy for cancer and people that get it.

So I'm just amazed that these things aren't...
Prof. Seyfried:
Well, the other thing you have to keep in mind is that the term *cure* has been a very reactive kind of term. We never use that term, we don't say "A metabolic therapy can cure cancer". What metabolic therapy can do is allow the patient to live longer. It's a management strategy.

You can manage the disease. Okay? In other words, you don't have to die so quickly. You can live a lot longer.

If you have cancer at your age - you look very healthy - suppose you get cancer and you manage it with metabolic therapy. And you die at 99 from a heart attack. Well, you obviously were cured from your cancer, because it didn't kill you.

But we don't know whether anybody is cured using metabolic therapy. All we know is that they seem to live longer than their were predicted with a higher quality of life. What's wrong with that? What is wrong with that scenario?
Dr. Chaffee:
Yes, and not being burned down by like the chemo and radiation!
Prof. Seyfried:
Yeah. I mean, let's be honest: Don't forget, we have millions of cancer survivors who have survived toxic radiation and chemo. But their body pays a significant price for that. They're suffering from
- gastrointestinal problems
- psychiatric problems
- hormonal imbalances
- microbiome disturbances

All kinds of things that make their life less enjoyable, less pleasurable. Because they were exposed to toxic poisons and toxic radiation.

This is stone age treatment, this should not happen in today's day and age. When we understand the biology of the disease very clearly. And yet, we're doing these crazy things to these poor people. It doesn't make any sense to me.

Dr. Chaffee:

I had a very good friend of mine that I grew up playing rugby with. And he unfortunately contracted sarcoma in his sinuses. Probably when he was in his late 30s, early 40s. A very fit guy, very active guy.

He went on and off, kept going... he struggled along with this for about three years: One of the chemo agents that he used just completely destroyed his nerves. He became almost crippled from this. Just from basically half a course of this chemotherapy.

And he stopped it! He just said... even though the cancer was responding well to it. He just said "Look, I don't want to survive cancer to be a cripple and an invalid. I'm not gonna take that anymore."

Prof. Seyfried:

Right. I have hundreds and hundreds of situations like this. Because I have thousands of people emailing me - and they always have a story.

What I feel so bad about is that they always contact me after they've been suffered through the standards of care. And their stories are horrific! I mean, you can't torture human beings as well as what some of the standard of care does to people.

I don't even think waterboarding would be as bad as some of the treatments they give these cancer patients. This is tragic! It's a tragedy of monumental proportions - and we don't have to do this!

Some of the chemotherapies our colleagues in Turkey use what we call a *metabolically supported chemotherapy:*

They use the lowest doses of chemo together with nutritional ketosis - which has really good outcomes. And they said they would prefer not to use any chemotherapy, but they're forced to do it by the system!

So the system of treatment seems to have permeated all healthcare industries in societies throughout the world. You go to India... I was shocked at how they love radiation over there, they radiate everybody over there. Any kind of a cancer.

I thought various cultures would be more open to metabolic therapy, but there seems to be a lock hold on cancer treatments throughout the world. They have to do this radiation and chemo. Now it's immunotherapy.

The problem with CAR-T immunotherapy... such a costly and very complicated therapy. What are they doing? Why are they doing this?

All they have to do is pull the plug on the glucose and glutamine, while under nutritional ketosis - and you don't have to spend 265,000 dollars to have your cancer managed! You see what I'm saying?

It comes right down to this whole concept of "What is cancer?

Is it a genetic disease? Or is it a mitochondrial metabolic disease?

And once you realize that it's a mitochondrial metabolic disease, most of the treatments we're doing to the cancer patients make no sense. They're not based on the fundamental underlying what the disease is.

So I don't know what I have what we have to do to get the word out. But somebody has to know about this. Otherwise, we're just going to continue to kill these poor patients, year in and year out.

Let's be honest.
Dr. Chaffee:
Yeah.
Prof. Seyfried:
I don't know what it is in Australia, in the United States alone, we have over 1,600 people dying every single day from cancer. Over 1,600.

When I was in China, it's 8,000! Because their population is large. As a matter of fact: In China, cancer has replaced heart disease as the number one killer of their population.
Dr. Chaffee:
Jesus!

Prof. Seyfried:
So what the hell is going on here?

And they're always saying "Oh, we're making major breakthroughs!" I ask where's the breakthroughs? With a breakthrough, the death rate should drop!

There's no breakthroughs. It's business as usual. More and more cancer deaths, no accountability.

I tell you, we're always running around, raising money for cancer patients. You know, *let's do the 5k run for breast cancer. Let's do this!*

What do they do with all the money that you get for raising? They give it to the people who think cancer's a genetic disease, keeping the system in place.

I mean, it's nuts. We got to start wizen up, people have to start asking "Where the hell is the accountability for the money that I'm raising?"

The only people who get healthy are the ones running and swimming to raise money for cancer research. You get healthy doing a bike ride – but with that money you're raising, you poison and irradiate the people that you're raising the money for!

It doesn't make any sense, does it?

Dr. Chaffee:
No, no. And that's the thing too, a good point that you raised: Cancer rates are getting worse. Like cancer eclipsing heart disease in China as the number one killer.

I looked at some of the gross figures in the US. I was looking at the numbers since we sort of overhauled our diet, after the 1977 USDA declaration that cholesterol is going to cause heart disease. And we reduced our fat and cholesterol intake by about 30%, reduced red meat by about 33%.

And we increase fruits and vegetables 30, 40%, increased carbs, increased sugar, all these things.

Since then, there's been roughly an overall tripling in cancer rates in the United States! You know, that cannot be genetic.

Prof. Seyfried:
No, no.

Dr. Chaffee:
Anyone who studies populations genetics knows very well that it's not possible to do that in a limited number of

generations. That means there's something in the environment that has changed and has affected this.

Prof. Seyfried:
Well, here's the other statistic that's often used to say *we're making major advances in cancer:*

The anti-smoking campaign that started probably around 1990, 1991...

Cancer was associated with smoking, so people stopped smoking. So if you use the 1991 rate of increase compared to today and you say "Look at how much how fewer cancer patients we have today!" - based on 1991 data.

Yeah, because everybody was smoking and dying in 1991! Not everyone, but many people were smoking and dying.

But if you look at the number of dead bodies accumulating every year, the number of dead bodies accumulate at the same percentage as the population growth.

So every year, the number of dead people from cancer goes up. The American Cancer Society has all the numbers, they all publish it every year. So this is a well documented event.

That numbers of dead people increase every year. Still: You don't use a 1991 rate to predict the success in the field!

"Oh, if we had continued to smoke in 2022, we would have had a lot more dead cancer deaths. „Of course you would, if people hadn't stopped smoking.

So the only real major advance we made was prevention – by the people. This had nothing to do with the science. We stopped smoking and therefore lung cancer numbers reduced.

And lung cancer is still the number one killer. But it would have killed a hell of a lot more if we hadn't stopped smoking.

But the treatments... you have to look at: Are there any new treatments that reduce cancer deaths? And the answer is *nope*. Zero! So it's a tragedy, no matter how you look at it.

Yet, the poor people in the hospital are suffering immensely, hair falling out... I say anytime you see a bald cancer patient, that person was treated by someone who doesn't understand the biology of the disease they're working on.

You shouldn't be bald, you're trying to kill cancer cells! What the hell? Why is your hair falling out? "Oh, the hair and the cancer cells share some common features - they're both growing."

But you don't want to kill all your good cells! Your gut cells, your hair cells, those have to be killed off? That tells me you have no idea.

Furthermore, they use these terms *precision medicine.* Well, how in the hell is your hair falling out with this so called precision medicine? Oh, it was "off target". if it's so precise - how come we have all these off-target effects on the person's body? I mean, this is such a bunch of crap.

When are they going to wise up to understand what's going on here. It just doesn't make any sense!

Dr. Chaffee:
Yeah, that's another thing, too. Something that you pointed out. In a cancer, like a tumor:

In medical school, obviously you get taught these genetic changes, and then this tumor just starts propagating. And all of the tumor cells should have the same DNA, monoclonal. But that's not what we see, we don't see that in tumors.

We see certain ones that have certain hallmarks and changes, increased mitosis. But a lot of these things just look normal they. They just look like normal tissue.

And yet, they behave as cancer. That to your point is: If these all have varying genetics, why are they all acting the same? That definitely looks like a downstream effect, as opposed to a causative effect.

Prof. Seyfried:
Oh yeah, absolutely! Absolutely. But everyone of the cells in that tumor is fermenting. They all have different genetic characteristics, but they're all fermenting.

So why are we so concerned about targeting the genetic mutations that differ in every single cell of the body - when the tumor cells are all fermenting?

That's the power of the somatic mutation theory. If the somatic mutation theory says *cancer is caused by genetic mutations*, mindlessly we go out and try to target all these different genetic mutations.

The mitochondrial metabolic theory says that they're all fermenting. The field has not yet accepted the mitochondrial metabolic theory as the origin of cancer, as Warburg had originally stated. They threw him under the bus.

When Watson and Crick first discovered the DNA structure, everybody ran off like the lemmings over the cliff, chasing DNA mutations. It's like the dog chasing his tail.

Now we've come to realize that all that genomic ideas, millions and billions of dollars spent on all this genomic stuff...

What we're finding, though - which is very interesting now - is that there are certain spontaneous mutations, that actually interfere with glucose and glutamine metabolism.

We call these *therapeutic mutations* - they're actually god's gift to the cancer patient by a rare event. Nobody knows. Like Pablo Kelly, he has an IDH1 mutation. It's called IDH1. This IDH1 mutation produces a metabolite called 2-hydroxyglutarate.

We and others have found that 2-hydroxyglutarate interferes with the glutamineolysis pathway, driving the energy of the tumor. And also the glycolysis pathway, building the raw material so the tumor can grow.

So the mutation itself is acting like a drug that can target two of the pathways driving the cancer. Can you believe this?

Dr. Chaffee:
Wow!

Prof. Seyfried:
And people that have this mutation are known to live twice as long as the people who don't have the mutation!

The problem is: Even the people with the mutation are given radiation and chemo, which reduces the ability of the very therapeutic mutation to work, it's unbelievable! (Laughs)

So if you don't do standard of care and are fortunate enough to have this therapeutic mutation, you can live a long time.

Pablo has this therapeutic mutation, goes on a carnivore / ketogenic diet. And every three years has had debulking surgery because this indolent tumor just hangs around. But he's never used the DON to target and kill off the rest of it.

So we have a strategy, I think. But it's really...

When you understand the biology of the disease, you can't help but be bewildered and overwhelmed by this new information - and how easy it is to get rid of cancer! Or manage it, let's put it that way. I wouldn't say get rid of it, but certainly manage it. It becomes a clear strategy.

It's just that more and more people need to know about this.

And once they know, there'll be a stampede for this.

Dr. Chaffee:

Yeah. What are some of the cancers that you found, that are more susceptible and sensitive to this metabolic treatment?

Prof. Seyfried:

Well, the alternative question is *which cancers have I found to be resistant*? Okay? This is because almost everyone is susceptible!

Every lung cancer that we've looked at, every breast, colon, bladder, kidney cancer - they're all very prone. They all have to ferment.

All the blood cancers are all driven by glutamine. So you're talking about all the major cancers.

You know, here's the situation: There are reports in the scientific literature, showing a genetically engineered mouse that has a genetically engineered lung cancer - that doesn't respond to metabolic therapy.

Now, the problem is, we don't know any human being walking around the planet, that has been genetically engineered the same way as this mouse has been genetically engineered. Nor does that person have a genetically engineered lung tumor.

Until we can find that person and ask that individual why they're not responding to metabolic therapy, I don't know.

But all of our mouse models that we found, all have naturally arising cancers. In other words: The cancer arose naturally in the natural host.

This is the best model that you can use because it's the same kind of cancer that would be found in dogs, a dog cancer arising naturally in the dog host. A human cancer arising naturally in the human host.

Those are the kinds of cancers that respond to metabolic therapy. Some of these genetically engineered things are not responsive in some ways. What reasons for, I have no clue.

I don't know why a mouse that's been so genetically engineered - with both the host and the cancer - doesn't respond to metabolic therapy. But I think I'll let somebody else figure that one out.

But who cares about that? Who gives a rat's ass about a mouse that's been genetically engineered, that doesn't respond to metabolic therapy? Right? Let's focus our attention on natural cancers.

Like dogs, for example: They respond remarkably well! Dogs with cancer. Cancer kills so many dogs. *It's like the number one killer of domestic dogs.*

The wolf never has rarely cancer. I don't think there's been a cancer in the literature, it must be very rare, in a wolf. Because they're eating natural, they're eating their natural diet in the wild. 105

They're not pounding down big burgers or jelly filled donuts, this kind of thing. And then, if you go to the zoo and ask the zookeeper "Why are you feeding your chimpanzees their natural diet? Why are giving them their natural diet? Why don't you let them eat jelly filled donuts and pizza, and drink Coca-Cola?"

What the zookeeper told me down here at the Franklin Park Zoo in Boston "Oh that would be animal cruelty. Animal abuse!" - and I'm saying "What the hell man! We're 98% similar to the chimpanzees, their DNA!" Right?

Let's take chimps and put them on an American diet from the time they're weaned. Let's take 100 chimps from the time they're weaning and give them only what we eat. Not their natural diet.

What do you think is going to happen?
- Cancer
- Dementia
- Type 2 diabetes
- Obesity

All the same sh*t that we have would be seen! But you can't do that because it's *animal abuse!*
Dr. Chaffee:
Yeah. Well, and that's it. They have the signs, saying "Do not feed the animals! This isn't their natural food!" They get very sick. And then we put that same nonsense into our mouths... and don't think that anything bad is going to happen.
Prof. Seyfried:
No, we get very, very sick! And the food industry and the pharmaceutical industry are both linked.

I had one of my students go and look at the investigation between the two organizations. Like, the big food industries producing all these foods that are poorly nutritious and full of highly processed carbs, that make you sick.

And on the other end of the other spectrum, the pharmaceutical companies will give you drugs and therapies to try to make you healthy.

Dr. Chaffee:
Yeah, exactly.

Prof. Seyfried:
What an industry! Right? It's unbelievable. It drives the economy... so I guess we have to be happy, because many of us are doing well - based on the revenue generation from these two industries overlapping with each other.

But I think that prevention is one thing. People who know about this certainly can...

Even Otto Warburg said *you can't get cancer if your mitochondria remain healthy*. And that's true, you can't get cancer if your mitochondria are healthy. That's prevention.

But we live in a society where it's hard not to eat. Okay, I saw you cooking the giant tomahawk rib eye. Well, I think that's wonderful and I would eat it - but also with a big baked potato, and a big loaf of bread with butter slathered all over it. And a big pile of unhealthy vegetables.

(Both laughing)

I mean, everybody would go down that path. But eating the tomahawk ribeye by itself... well, I don't know about that. But I certainly would do something like that.

Dr. Chaffee:
Yeah, that's funny... I was gonna say, too...

One of the things I thought, exactly as you said, is that we don't see cancers in wild animals - and we don't see them in the zoo. Everyone says that "Well, animals in the wild, they probably don't live long enough to get cancer." But that never explains animals in the zoo. Or "They're active and they're running around."

But an animal in the zoo is sitting around its whole life - and they don't get these cancers. The cancer rates in dogs and cats,

these have all increased dramatically since the inception of packaged dog and cat food.
Prof. Seyfried:
Yeah, yeah, absolutely. And the zoos maintain a very nutritious diet, they have a staff of veterinarians that monitor the diet. They're so carefully monitored, these zoo primates, the gorillas and the chimps, are monitored very carefully. All the time, in regards to nutritional balances.

That's why they said, if we gave them jelly filled donuts and pizza, they would get hammered.

There is a family of chimps that live with humans, they're on the web. It's a group of chimps that live with humans. You should see these chips go wild when they get the jelly sandwiches! They're banging on the table, they're getting all excited eating jelly sandwiches.
Dr. Chaffee:
That's awful!
Prof. Seyfried:
Haha! Yeah, you can go on the web, there's a bunch of chimps that live with a human family. And while they talk, the chimps are pounding down all this stuff. Loving it, banging on the table...
Dr. Chaffee:
...Captain Crunch, just going after it...
Prof. Seyfried:
I mean, who wouldn't? You could drop off your box of donuts into the pen with the chimps down there, they'd be all over the donuts. And the other guys that weren't getting the donuts would be all upset.

It just shows you that we as a species have used technology,,, sweetness in our evolutionary past was only rare and seasonal. But our technology has now made it permanent.

Now we can get this sweet stuff all the time - and we like it! We evolved to like sweets. So everything has been carefully developed, tweaked, to all of our taste buds, to make us want to eat more of this. Even though we put ourselves at risk for cancer, dementia, heart disease, diabetes, all this kind of stuff.

We're willing to still eat the foods that are putting us in that situation, because they taste so good.

Dr. Chaffee:
And to your previous point about this unholy alliance between food and pharmacy:

Dr. Robert Lustig of UCSF, he mentioned in one of his books - if I can remember the numbers correctly – that the sugar industry makes about 1.3 trillion dollars a year, gross figures.

And what we spend just treating the metabolic issues that are derived from sugar consumption is about 2.4 trillion dollars! So this is a massive, massive amount of money. I mean, that's the entire federal budget, just spent on eating and supporting sugar addiction.

Prof. Seyfried:
Yeah, of course. But if a politician came out and said

"Listen, our health industry budget is crippling our nation. It's actually causing a crisis, putting us at risk. So we're all going to go back and do Paleolithic eating! We're going to eat tomahawk rib eyes, we're going to cut down on our carcinogenic vegetables..."

How long do you think that guy's going to remain in office? They'll vote his ass out right away!

But when you have the cancer, then all of a sudden your whole world begins to change, *how come I wasn't told about this?!*

Well, we're telling you now! Do you want to make the choice or not?

Dr. Chaffee:
So with glioblastoma: In your animal models, what are you finding to be the results when you put them on this, the DON and the restrictive dietary ketosis. How much of a benefit are you seeing in those mice?

Prof. Seyfried:
Oh yeah, we're getting 3, 4 times longer survival.

Dr. Chaffee:
Wow!

Prof. Seyfried:
One of the things we've done... because we took these glioblastoma cells and we identified the metastatic cancer as being a type of plastic macrophage.

And in the GBM, if you look at glioblastoma, many of the so-called mesenchymal cells, the cells that have this mesenchymal phenotype, are the most highly invasive.

They did call it glioblastoma multiforme, because of all the different kinds of cells that you would see in there. The mesenchymal kind of cell is the most invasive.

And when we took those cells out of the brain of the mouse and put them in the flank, they metastasized. They spread all over the body.

Then we found out that all metastatic cancers have macrophage characteristics. So we know the nature of the metastatic cell: It's a type of a macrophage - and it loves glutamine and glucose.

When we put them in the flank, they spread all over the body. We use bioluminescence imaging, we can image the tumor cells and see how much they've spread through the body.

Then... we call them *terminal mice*. They're going to die in a couple of days. You can see the heavy breathing, you can see their immobility.

Then we hit him with our diet drug cocktail - and within 3 or 4 days, these guys are back, walking around like they never had anything! They still have cancer, but it's been managed.

So: We took these guys from death's doorstep... normally they would be dead by 30 days if we did nothing. Or if we would just continue to feed them the high carbohydrate standard lab chow.

But then, we got them now to live over 4 and a half months! 5 times longer than they normally would have.

We haven't published this yet, but we plan to publish it. Once we have all the conditions of the drug / diet cocktails defined.

We're seeing it for pediatric cancer in the mice, too. Because we're doing the same thing to these little kids that we do to the adults. We hit them with high-dose chemo, we hit them with high radiation. We do the same toxic things to those little kids as we do to adults.

And we can take these pediatric models that we've developed here at Boston College, and... We can keep these mice alive so much longer and in such a higher quality of life!

We know that we can get the same results in the pediatric clinic as we see with these natural pediatric brain tumors in in the mice. We know we can keep people alive with advanced metastatic cancer, if we do drug diet cocktails at the right time. Don't interfere with this!

Don't forget: With none of our mice, we do radiation [The groups that get metabolic therapy]. So the results that we get... They say "Oh, you just get all those great results in the mice, you wouldn't see that in the human."

Well, maybe - because we don't irradiate the mice! So if we'd radiate the mice, maybe we'll see what we get in the human. I don't know because we don't plan to do that. And I don't plan to irradiate, why?

Now, I'm not saying radiation is bad for everything. Because I think, if you have a tumor in a particular location, it's well defined, it's not metastatic – then, radiation could potentially cure that kind of a tumor. So we don't want to throw all these things under the bus.

We did temozolomide with metabolic therapy, and we showed that it was no better than... Temozolomide is the primary chemo for brain cancer.

We showed that it was no better than metabolic therapy, used with hyperbaric oxygen.

And the mice never got sick with our metabolic therapy. They got sick with the temozolomide. So we tried Temozolomide with metabolic therapy: We put them all together.

Yeah, they did good, but they didn't do any better than metabolic therapy by itself - without the sickness!

So I'm saying: Why are we doing all this stuff? Why are we doing what we're doing? Because Temozolomide generates huge revenue for the hospital!

Dr. Chaffee:
Yeah.

Prof. Seyfried:
So we're not interested in the revenue generation here, we're interested in how long we can keep animals alive, with metastatic advanced stage 4 cancers. We have a different outcome, different perspective on looking at this whole thing.

But yeah, we have achieved levels of success that are beyond anything we would have ever expected. Without toxicity! And that's diet drug cocktails, that will work just great.

We published a big paper on this, called *The Press Pulse Therapeutic Strategy*, with some of my clinician colleagues. It outlines the framework for how we would treat human cancers with the press pulse therapeutic strategy.

The diet is the press - and then we use strategic drugs, with the diet, to pulse them. Not chronically use them, but pulse the drugs. And that slowly degrades the tumor, while enhancing the health and vitality of the normal cells.

Many cancer patients who come into the clinic, they not only have cancer, they often have diabetes, they often have some other comorbidities associated with the fact that they have cancer.

In our metabolic press pulse strategies, we not only manage the cancer, reducing it significantly. But we also get rid of the diabetes, we get rid of the hypertension, we get rid of the other comorbidities that these patients also have had.

Clearly: Linking all of these chronic diseases to a common underlying provocative situation - which is nutritional imbalance. Diets and treatments that provoke the growth of these tumors, and persist on these kinds of conditions.

So clearly, once you understand the biology of the problem, the solutions become much, much more clear and logical.

Dr. Chaffee:
Yeah. I was going to say, too, about the radiation: Obviously, we do use this in the pediatric populations. It can be absolutely devastating to those kids.

I think that if I were in a position... even not knowing the things that we're talking about now. I don't think I would ever let my child get radiation for a tumor.

Prof. Seyfried:
You might not have a choice.

Dr. Chaffee:
What?

Prof. Seyfried:
You might not have a choice! Because if that child is lower than 16 years of age or 18, the system determines what you should do to that child.

Dr. Chaffee:
Oh, really?

Prof. Seyfried:

The system determines. The parents are taken out of the equation. Unless... Remember, the woman that went to Mexico to save the life of her child?

The system controls what you do to that child. So even if you said *the standard of care involves radiation and chemo for that child*, it's very hard to break the system. They'll have you arrested as 'parental neglect'.

That's what I'm talking about: The system is very powerful.

Dr. Chaffee:

That's definitely too much! I've seen kids who have grown up after getting radiation like this, it completely stuns their mental development. So where wherever were, it probably damaged them from that point...

Say, they're three, they damaged them from three - and then they never develop past that.

So you have this person in this 30-year old body, with the mind of a 5-year-old. Or less. And it's absolutely tragic to see that.

Prof. Seyfried:

More tragic is: It doesn't have to happen!

Dr. Chaffee:

Yeah, exactly.

Prof. Seyfried:

That doesn't have to happen, that's the tragedy. That child could have been rescued. I'm not saying the child could have been cured, but if the child lives to be the same age, they would be cognitively intact. Not cognitively challenged.

Dr. Chaffee:

Yeah, and we talk about quality of life and we do give people the choice:

Is this something that you want to do? Given the fact that this is going to be a pretty rough road. Do you want to just live out your last months at a better standard of living? Or go for the gold?

I think that especially when you're talking about a child who could potentially have such devastating damage to their brain and their development, for me, I would never want that personally - and I don't think I would ever want that for my child either.

Prof. Seyfried:
No, no one does. But this is the way it is. And you often see the child...

They're given such high dose steroids, they get the big moon face. The steroids are driving blood sugars to extremely high levels. Then once you see that phenotype, the big moon face – whether it's in a child or an adult with a glioblastoma – you know they're finished.

You know that the therapy itself is killing those people. That's the tragedy.

What I just said to you, that statement that I just made, is not known to the majority of practitioners in the field: They are under the impression that this is helping their patient! This is the gap in knowledge that needs to be closed.

We cannot continue to do this toxic therapy on these poor people. Whether it's a child or an adult. It speaks to the lack of knowledge on the part of the field treating a disease. Okay?

It has to change. It has to change, otherwise we have to continue to see these tragedies one after another. Not only in America, throughout the world. You're in Australia, they're doing the same thing down there as we do here. In England, Germany, Japan. They're all doing the same thing.

It's a worldwide tragedy! And it will only change once everybody comes to realize that cancer is a mitochondrial metabolic disease. We could make a dent in this disease so quick, if people knew what I just said.

The problem is: They don't want to know about it, they don't want to hear about it, they don't want to talk about it. For various reasons.

Dr. Chaffee:
On that note: You mentioned there are some clinics and centers that are using this as a model. Where are these guys at and how are they getting away with it?

Prof. Seyfried:
Well, I think there's small clinics that have patients... they have to be offered an alternative. Right now, if you go to the main hospitals like Dana-Farber, MD Anderson, Sloan Kettering, wherever else they have these major cancer centers, they're not offering metabolic therapy.

Doctors should offer metabolic therapy, see with the patients. The problem is: If you're going to be Dana-Farber or MD Anderson and you want to do metabolic therapy - there's no one there really that knows what to do!

You have to have a staff of professionals that know what to do, and how to do it! Okay? Without that knowledge base, it's not going to work.

Even worse: The young people going through medical schools in the oncology area, *they're not trained to do metabolic therapy.* So where is the training coming from?

We have written a protocol to treat cancer patients, based on metabolic therapy. With Miriam Kalamian, a world-renowned expert on keto for cancer and diet for this. She's helped a lot of cancer patients.

We wrote a treatment protocol. Can it be used? It will not be used in the major hospitals, of course. Because you're doing it as an alternative to radiation, chemo, immunotherapies and these other kinds of things.

But it can be done in smaller clinics. In smaller clinics that are not so yoked by the system, to do what they have to do.

The goal is to keep people alive - and have the people themselves tell everyone *this is what I did.* Guy Tenenbaum, he's on the web, overcame his stage 4 prostate cancer using metabolic approaches!

So you're getting more and more vocal advocates that are telling others that, "Listen, do metabolic therapy!" Now, is it easy? I don't want to let people think that doing metabolic therapy is a cakewalk.

Because a lot of the success rides on your shoulders: How compliant are you to not eat carbohydrates - which can be very hard for a lot of people.

Dr. Chaffee:

Yeah. That's one of the things I see in clinic, here in neurosurgery: We get these people with the GBMs, this devastating diagnosis.

I think every single patient that I've ever done a consultation with... and we do this once a week, we have everyone come in with all the new diagnoses. And I don't think there's a single person that hasn't asked me "Okay, what can *I* do? How can *I* do this?" They don't want to feel helpless, but it is just out of their control.

And I remember getting really upset at another physician. They asked him, sort of "Well, should I stop eating sugar? Should I stop drinking alcohol? Or what should I do?" - and the doctor's like "You know what? You probably don't have that long anyway, so just do whatever you want." I was so furious at that!

Prof. Seyfried:
Yeah.

Dr. Chaffee:
The person looked so defeated, he was like "Yeah, I guess it just doesn't matter." I was like "Of course it matters! It absolutely matters! You have control, you have a say in this. You have a dog in this fight, you are able to affect your own course of your life!"

And just seeing their eyes, literally hope just rising in their eyes... and I try to mitigate that because this isn't good any way you cut it.

But I tell them: I tell them about your work, I point them in the direction of your material and studies, and I just say:

"Hey look, I'm not telling you that this is going to cure anything, it's not going to stop anything. But there's a lot of evidence that says that if you do this, this will help. Here, just go to the source.

See what you think.

Prof. Seyfried:
You're 100% correct about that and I can't emphasize that more than what you just said. Because I see people... once they understand about the glucose ketone index, measuring their own blood every day - not every day, but every other day or whatever, using a little meter.

And they're collecting the numbers and they know what direction those numbers have to go, for that therapy to be effective – with that, they get really motivated!

They now know that they are able to do something. They are in control of their own destiny. And they work very hard and they become extremely motivated!

This is what Pablo did: When he knew what numbers he had to achieve in order to put pressure on the growth of that tumor, he knew he was in control.

You give the patient now power, they have the power and they get motivated to know what they need to do. You're absolutely right: Nobody should ever be told there's nothing more we can do.

Especially at the beginning of their disease. Then they have to know that it's a long haul. It's not like *I'm really good at this for a month.*

No, no. You're gonna have to bite the bullet on this and power it through, until you have achieved control of that growth. The growth does not control you, control the growth of the cancer

Dr. Chaffee:

Yeah!

Prof. Seyfried:

The patient can do that with the proper motivation, with the proper training. So I can't emphasize more what you just said. You've got to let these patients know that they're part of the fight and they can control this.

You'd be surprised how much longer these people live, in a higher quality of life. And when they... I don't want to say they all pass. But I've had people tell me, or their loved ones, told me that "This guy fought the fight. He felt so good about himself - and even though he may not have made it all the way, he lived 2, 3 times longer than he was supposed to live - at a much higher quality of life! And never had to suffer and die in these painful situations."

Then there's many people who are still fighting the fight and should have died a long time ago, and they're still on!

If I had the drugs that work with the diet, we would be able to settle this in a much more defined period of time. So yeah, there's a lot of hope for the future.

I would say the future of cancer is bright, not bleak! You know, it's a whole new strategy and I think that the future of cancer is: We can keep this disease managed and people are going to emerge in a healthier state and feel much better about themselves.

That's my view. I base it on my understanding of the biology of the disease, and 30 years of research in the field, looking at this problem. And publishing all these papers. This is the way I see it. I think the future is far brighter than it should be, than people make it out to be.

Dr. Chaffee:

Yeah, good! I agree with you! Just trying to get this out there and let people know that they actually have a say in this. hen they can actually affect the course of this disease. They're not just out of control and just at the whims of the chemo and radiation - but they actually have something to say in this as well.

When did you get this focus in your line of research? I know that when you were at Yale, you were doing research on seizures and preventing seizures with ketosis.

Which is something that I've looked into. And it's like, we've been using this for nearly 90 years to treat refractory seizures. But yet, it's something that almost no neurologist that I know of uses. I've seen a lot of people with epilepsy, have spoken to them. I always ask them *have they ever spoken to you about your diet?* Not a single one has said yes.

Which just blows my mind! Because it's such a simple thing. It may not be easy to implement, but it is straightforward, and it has a lot of evidence behind it.

Prof. Seyfried:

Well, don't forget: At that time, Yale was one of the leaders in the field of epilepsy research. Gilbert Glaser was the chair of the department. Had written many, many distinguished books and papers on epilepsy.

And they told me... because I was working on ganglioside biochemistry at the time, looking at different disorders of lipid metabolism. But they said: "If you want to stay at Yale, you better work on something to do with epilepsy."

So we were mapping genes for epileptic seizures. Everybody was excited mapping genes. Because the idea was if you map the gene, you could figure out the product and you can make a treatment for that product.

Then I realized that we always tried to do the same kind of chemicals and things all the time - why don't we try keto? I didn't do ketogenic diet until I came to Boston.

I tried to get a grant at Yale, but they said *nobody's interested in ketogenic diets for epilepsy, we have all these drugs.* But then Jim Abrams of the movie industry, produced the film *First do no harm* with Meryl Streep - his son Charlie had epilepsy. He started the Charlie Foundation.

He brought together a lot of people in the epilepsy field to look at: Why are we not using ketogenic diets to manage epilepsy, when it was known since by 1921 by Wilder at Mayo Clinic? Why are we not doing this?

So one of my students went out to the meeting, we were still doing looking at epilepsy. She came back and said "Hey listen! We should put our mice on ketogenic diets!" And sure enough... we had mapped all these genes, but the thing was the diet blocked the seizures. It was really quite an interesting thing.

Then calorie restriction was even more powerful, along with ketogenic diets. And then we were working on the gangliosides for brain cancer, we were doing a lot of work on brain cancer.

Then we said "Why don't we see if the diet works on brain cancer?" After the results, I said "Oh my god, this is unbelievable! What's going on here?!" Then we discovered Otto Warburg had said this many, many years ago.

We know that the tumors can't burn ketones for energy because their mitochondria are defective, they need glucose. So when the glucose is low and the ketones are elevated, the tumors shrink. Makes perfect sense, Otto Warburg was right!

That then send us off into a better understanding of how we manage cancer metabolically, coming from our understanding of how ketogenic diets work on epileptic seizures.

Actually, we still don't know the mechanism by which ketogenic diets block epilepsy, because it's a very complicated brain wiring scenario that has to be looked into. But it became crystal clear as how this diet could stop cancer growth, or restrict cancer growth.

The fact is that we have tens of thousands of little kids around the world, using ketogenic diets every day to manage their seizures. Yet, when you talk about it in cancer, they go "Oh, it could hurt the kid, it could hurt the patient! The toxic effects of ketogenic diets,"

Are you kidding me? We have thousands of little kids doing ketogenic diets for epilepsy, and nobody's talking about that - but when you take a little kid with cancer *oh no, terribly toxic, it's nutritionally imbalanced...*

What? Are you nuts? Compared to radiation and chemo? You're telling me that a ketogenic diet is more harmful than radiation and chemo? I mean, give me a break

Dr. Chaffee:
Exactly!

Prof. Seyfried:
This is the absurdity of dealing with the field. We came to this state where we are through a long, circuitous path. Not knowing where any of this would have ever taken us. But we were aware enough of the underlying mechanisms of action to know what we were doing, why we were doing it, and how it works.

Now the big challenge is getting the word out to people and seeing more and more success stories of using this. Now in Los Angeles, a colleague of mine has a big trial with ketogenic diet for glioblastoma.

And he's getting spectacular results, more than he would have ever imagined. But that's still with upfront standard of care! He and I know... I said "If you took away that radiation and chemo, your results would probably be even more spectacular."

So it just takes time for the system to come to adjust and realize what's happening here. There is a very clear mechanism of action. So it just takes time, that's all.

But I feel that this current time is being wasted, and we're sacrificing all these poor kids and adults to cancer, that's the tragedy. That this doesn't have to happen and yet, it's happening.

Dr. Chaffee:
So these damaged mitochondria: Obviously, this is precipitating this issue. Can that ever reverse? Or is there always be a point of no return... but does that ever come back? Meaning the status of healthy mitochondria.

Prof. Seyfried:
Well, that was one of the big things that I did when I bundled together all the nuclear mitochondrial transfer experiments that were done in animal systems over decades.

All independent of each other, done by some of the best developmental biologists in the field, and I spoke to some of these individuals.

If you take the nucleus of the tumor cell that has all the mutations that are supposedly drivers, and you drop that nucleus into a new cytoplasm, you get growth regulation! Not growth dysregulation.

And sometimes you can form a whole frog or a mouse from the nucleus of a tumor cell. So you replaced essentially the bad mitochondria. In other words you put that nucleus into a cytoplasm with fresh mitochondria - and those new mitochondria are able to re-regulate the growth and development.

Despite the continued presence of the so-called driver gene mutations that we're supposed to... I mean, this is the hardest evidence against this gene theory.

If you do the reverse, if you take the normal nucleus and drop it into a cytoplasm that has cancerous mitochondria, the cell will either die or form dysregulated cancer cells. This is clear evidence. Getting back to your question: *Can we revert cancer by putting new mitochondria in there.* It's called mitochondrial therapy, actually. I think that's gonna come in the future.

I think it's so new that eventually we will be able to maybe replace them. But I don't want to, at this point, say "Let's see if we can restore the growth regulation of a cancer cell by putting in new mitochondria."

I think it's better at this point to kill them off, get rid of them! Put them in a growth lock hold, rather than trying to re-educate them. I think mitochondrial therapy for the future is going to be really exciting and interesting.

I don't think we're there yet. So let's work with what we can do, and make a real big difference. Then we'll move forward with these newer kinds of therapies for the future.

But right now, let's just put a lock hold on these cancer cells and keep people alive in a healthier state. If that means eating tomahawk ribeyes, I think you'll find a number of people that would buy on to that.

Dr. Chaffee:
Yeah. That experiment that you spoke of, taking the nucleus and then putting it into a new cytoplasm and the mitochondria - showing that you have all these genetic changes and it doesn't behave as cancer. And you take the mitochondria and put them in - and it does behave as cancer! That's qed, as far as I'm concerned.

Prof. Seyfried:
Yeah, but it's still...

The response by the oncology field is: They don't want to talk about it, they don't want to look at it and they don't want to hear about it!

That's because it's so devastating to an entire industry. That, once that becomes more widely recognized...

Dr. Chaffee:
Yeah.

Prof. Seyfried:
...and it's been repeated over and over, in all different kinds of models. So what's the holdup? What is the holdup here?

Somebody has to scratch their head and say "What? Why do we continue to persist with therapies, that put patients at risk for all kinds of health diseases, when we have a solution, a better approach, to management than we currently have?" What is the holdup here? [Laughter] **Dr. Chaffee:**
So if someone were to have cancer now, what would be the best way to manage it? Obviously, going ketogenic or even carnivore. What ratio are they looking for to get?

Like, what is so the best way for people to manage this at home, if they don't have access to one of these clinics that are popping up?

Prof. Seyfried:
Well, as I said in the letters that I sent to people, I'm not a physician. I can't tell you what to do and what not to do.

All I can do is provide you with information, knowledge, from published papers and observations. And I'll let the physicians in the clinics treat the patients.

We know what we need to do, see the press pulse paper. Now, a lot of people cannot do water-only fasting because it's too much of a shock. The brain is addicted to glucose. And it's just as difficult to get off glucose than it is to get off heroin, alcohol and nicotine, these kinds of things.

But the body can adjust to the change. So, you will have withdrawal symptoms. What we realized is that if the patient were to gradually transition to a zero carbohydrate diet, for several weeks - even that can be difficult for some patients...

But it's not as much of a jump to doing a water-only fast. I tried it, man! Going cold turkey on carbs is really, really tough! I mean, you can smell stuff cooking like blocks away.

Dr. Chaffee:
Haha!

Prof. Seyfried:
It's unbelievable! It's too hard. What we've learned is that patients can transition to water-only fasting after a couple of weeks on zero carb diets. With meat, no carbs at all. Some vegetables, we're not as opposed to veggies as you might be.

But if we can get organically grown vegetables... grow them in your backyard, using manure and these kinds of things.

I tell you, then the transition to water-only fasting for a few days is way easier. Bring those blood sugars down, bring the ketones up. Get into the new diet state, then you hit him with the drugs. A drug like DON and some of the other drugs.

There are all these parasite medications. Man, they're really damn powerful!

Yeah, you hit them with **Mebendazole, Fenbendazole**, they target some of the metabolic pathways that the cancer cells need.

Dr. Chaffee:
Okay!

Prof. Seyfried:
All this stuff is cheap. Now here's the interesting thing...

And Bendazole was really cheap, it's a parasite medication. For some sort of worms. You can get the pills over in India for 50 cents a tablet.

But now, when we realized in the United States these medications work with cancer treatment, it's 300 dollars a tablet!

Dr. Chaffee:
Aww! Come on!

Prof. Seyfried:
Yeah, you tell me what's the drive in this industry. It's not helping, it's revenue generation.

You know the guy Martin Shkreli, the most hated man in America? Who made the EpiPens like 800 dollars?

Dr. Chaffee:
Right!

Prof. Seyfried:
Remember that guy? He took advantage of the system because he could. Everybody hated the guy.

But the pharmaceutical industry does the same thing, they just don't broadcast it. It's now called shkreli, *you shkreli the price* of all these things you can make a buck on.

Dr. Chaffee:
Haha!

Prof. Seyfried:
It's terrible, right? It's really despicable behavior.

Dr. Chaffee:
It is!

Prof. Seyfried:
Yeah, but that's the business of America.

These are the drugs. You can get drugs on the cheap, as long as know how to use them. You put them together with diet drug combinations, and you can get a really good powerful management of cancer.

But you have to have knowledgeable people. They have to know doses, timing and scheduling. This is all quite doable, the framework is already here, we published the framework. So, if people are willing to know how to do this, they're willing to take it, they should follow that framework.

Cancer patients, sure, they can do a lot of it themselves - as long as they're educated and told what to do and how to do it.

Then you have non-invasive imaging technology that can monitor their cancer, to see whether or not it's growing. Whether or not it's stabilized - or whether or not it's still there or not.

We don't need to be taking punch biopsies and doing all this crazy stuff. What are you doing biopsies for?

Everybody's like "Oh, I gotta have a biopsy of my cancer." Why? "I don't know if it's malignant." Well, if it's malignant, you should never take a punch biopsy, you could spread it all over the damn body!

And if it's a benign, what the are hell you sticking a benign tumor for? So they want to get a gene profile of the cells that come out of your tumor - to tell you what kind of a new drug, a new toxic drug, that will target that mutation you should take.

But: The damn cells are using glucose and glutamine! Why don't you target that before you stick the tumor?!

I mean, everything we're doing is like back ass forward. You got to know what to do, how to do it. Educate people, educate the practitioners - and things will begin to change. They have to change, we can't continue to do what we're doing.

Dr. Chaffee:
I completely agree. Professor Seyfried, thank you so much for coming on. I really appreciate it, it's been an absolute pleasure to speak with you.

I've been referencing your work and pointing people towards you for a number of years now. I really appreciate this opportunity to speak with you, so thank you very much!

Prof. Seyfried:
Well, thank you. I hope some of this information can help people.

And our support that we have comes from philanthropy and private foundations.

Obviously, there are people who recognize what we are doing, what we are saying and the strategies.

There are good people! Who say *you're doing the right thing let me support what you're doing.* Because it's very hard to get the federal government granting system funds, through the National Cancer Institute - when everybody thinks cancer is a genetic disease. And you're coming along, telling them "It's not!"

You don't go very far in getting funds for doing that kind of stuff. But yeah, we'll keep pushing. We have the best pre-clinical model systems, the best trained staff a knowledgeable staff - and we're not going anywhere.

Dr. Chaffee:
Good!

Prof. Seyfried:
We're pushing forward on this until the job is done. So thanks for reading, I hope this helps your audience.

Dr. Chaffee:
Well, I hope it does too. And there are certainly people that are suffering from cancer or they will become afflicted by it. I think

anyone who reads this and knows someone with cancer, I really encourage them to borrow them this book - so that they can really understand what's going on.

Actually, so that they can really understand, that they have a lot more to say in their own prognosis and recovery than they might think they do!

Professor Seyfried, what's the best place for people to find you and find your work? You mentioned your email that you send out to people. Is there a link to a website or something?

Prof. Seyfried:

Yes, there's a link to the **Foundation For Cancer Metabolic Therapies**, we obtain money from private foundations.

People can also support us through **Boston College**, they can send funds directly to my research program.

Dr. Chaffee:

Okay!

Prof. Seyfried:

These kinds of things. And believe it or not, more and more people are coming out to support this. Because it's going to have a greater impact in supporting almost anything else in the cancer field, there's no question about that.

So the faster we get our papers published, the more evidence we continue to accumulate... case reports, human case reports: We do that!

So I help the physicians to write up the case reports on the patients that have survived longer than would be expected. It takes a lot of my time, of course, but I'm willing to do this.

And our peer-reviewed scientific publications continue to push this field forward.

This requires funding to do because we have to pay lots of things. There's animal costs, staff costs, consumables. Things that we use, equipment costs, things to maintain...

Bottom line is: Yeah, I send a letter out that has information, helps cancer patients make decisions, try to get them with the right contacts. People who understand what's going on, and then they take it from there.

This has been the plan so far. It seems to be gaining more and more momentum, as more and more word gets out about this whole cancer thing. And things begin to change.

Dr. Chaffee:
Fantastic! I encourage people to go, visit and to donate. I think that this sort of work is really important.

Prof. Seyfried:
The letters that I send out... it's only asking for a donation if you feel that that information helps you. If something helps you, you might consider a donation. I am not asking anybody... only if the information that I send is of value. I don't charge anything for this.

The bottom line is to see the results, more than anything else. I think that's the most important thing at this stage.

Dr. Chaffee:
I completely agree. There's a lot of things that I don't get paid for as well. I stay late, talk to people. And talk to people outside of the hospital, to try and get them better.

Because that's why we're here! You know, I think a lot of people, a lot of doctors and researchers are still in that mindset - but unfortunately, some have forgotten that. Or forgotten that it's even possible to do that anymore.

Prof. Seyfried:
Yeah. Anyway, I'll let you go. Thank you very much and thank you for the interview.

Dr. Chaffee:
Thank you, I really appreciate it.

Other Summary Books

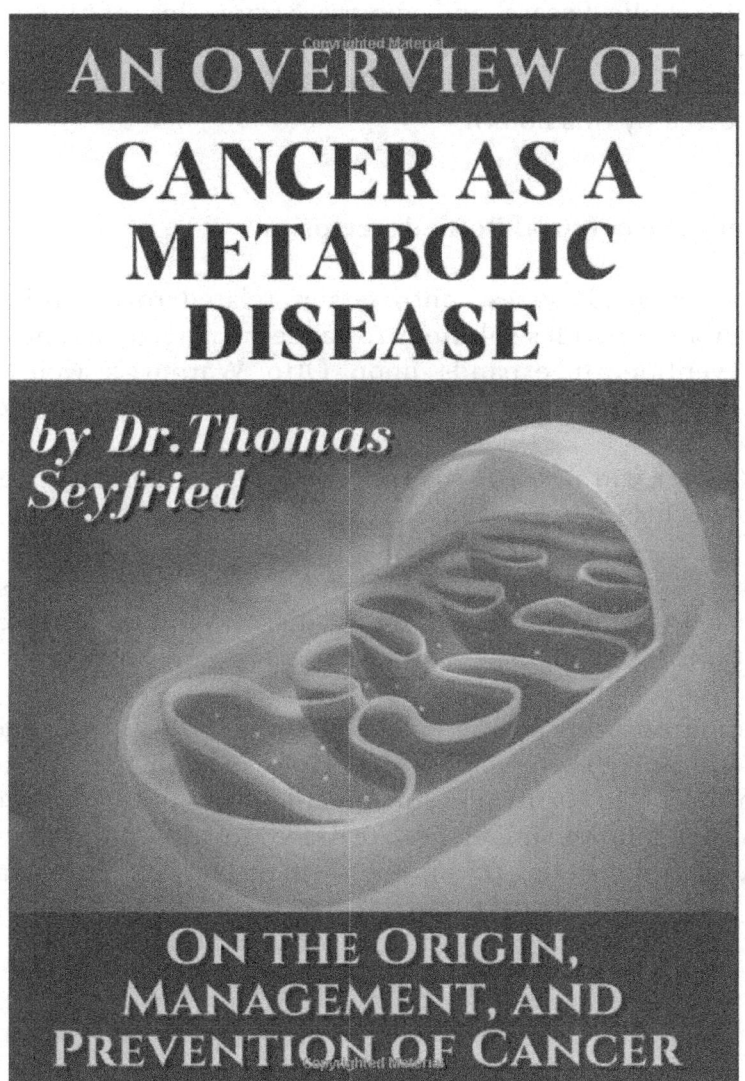

25% of the royalties of this book will be donated to Dr. Seyfrieds research!

<u>This research will actually make a REAL impact, as it studies the real causes and treatment opportunities of cancer!</u>

This book is a summary of Dr. Thomas Seyfrieds book "Cancer as a metabolic disease" and comprises transcripts of his talks and interviews, as well as texts by his collegue Dr. Dominic D'Agostiono and Travis Christofferson (whose foundation will be supported by this book).

Here the original Book description:

The book addresses controversies related to the origins of cancer and provides solutions to cancer management and
prevention. It expands upon Otto Warburg's well-known theory that all cancer is a disease of energy metabolism. However,
Warburg did not link his theory to the "hallmarks of cancer" and thus his theory was discredited.

This book aims to provide evidence, through case studies, that cancer is primarily a metabolic disease requring metabolic solutions for its management and prevention.

Support for this position is derived from critical assessment of current cancer theories. Brain cancer case studies are presented as a proof of principle for metabolic solutions to disease management, but similarities are drawn to other types of cancer, including breast and colon, due to the same cellular mutations that they demonstrate.

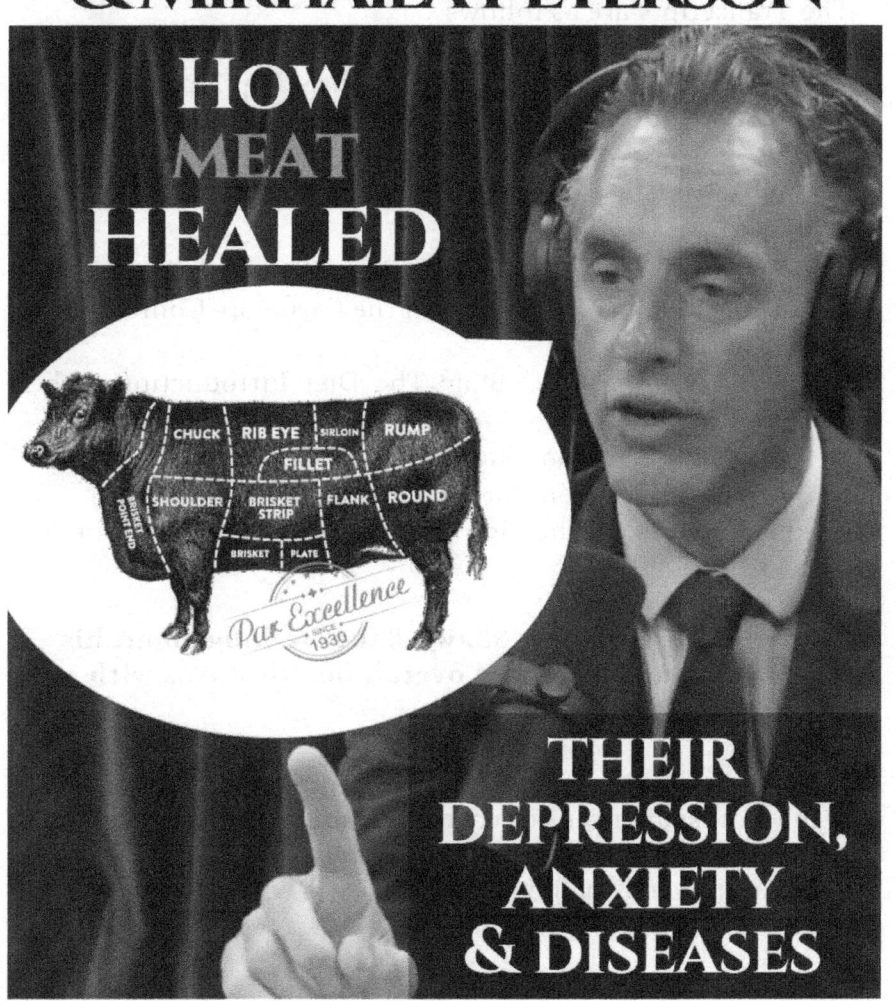

The book offers 11 Chapters of revised transcripts of Dr. Jordan Peterson & Mikhaila Peterson on:

- how they cured their disease, depression and health issues with the carnivore diet and
- how ill people could start this kind of eating as well.

The Transcripts are as follows:

1. The Agenda with Steve Paikin Digesting Depression
2. Joe Rogan Podcast 1070
3. Joe Rogan Podcast 1139
4. Podcast Interview of Mikhaila Peterson with Robb Wolf, including blood work
5. Podcast Interview with Ivor Cummins
6. Talk by Mikhaila Peterson at the Carnivore Conference in Boulder, 2019
7. Mikhaila Petersons Blog: The Diet Introduction of her Lion Diet on YouTube
8. Mikhaila Peterson: Should you start an elimination diet?
9. Mikhaila Peterson: Jordan Peterson's Lion Diet
10 Mikhaila Peterson: The Lion Diet (Introduction of her diet on YouTube

11. Bonus-Transcript: Dr. Shawn Baker talking about his coronary calcium score and overall health status with years of being carnivore.

The transcriptions are revised, which means that the grammar and the wordsequences got corrected, adding phrases here and there, as well as leaving out other elements that hinder understanding and the joy of reading.

Sources

Chapter

1) Text (editors revised transcription) & slides based on YT video:

Channel: „ Anthony Chaffee MD "

Channel-Url: https://www.youtube.com/@anthonychaffeemd

Title: " Why We Are Carnivores Slide Presentation, with Dr Anthony Chaffee"

Video-Url: https://www.youtube.com/watch?v=C-WUb3mJEs0

2) Text based on Youtube video: Same channel and Channel URL

Title: " Carnivore For Beginners: How To Start A Carnivore Diet with Tips, Tricks, and Common Pitfalls"

Video-Url: https://www.youtube.com/watch?v=V8ns1j28vhc

3) Text (editors revised transcription) & slides based on YT video:

Channel: „ Low Carb Down Under "

Channel-Url: https://www.youtube.com/@lowcarbdownunder

Title: " Dr. Anthony Chaffee - 'Plants are trying to kill you!' "

Video-Url: https://www.youtube.com/watch?v=j1cqNDDG4aA

4) Text based on YT video: Same channel and Channel URL as 1)

"The Hard Facts about Cancer and Diet with Prof. Thomas Seyfried…"
Video-Url: https://www.youtube.com/watch?v=1ebPZP9hBPA

Thanks to Dr. Anthony Chaffee for his important work to cure people
of our modern diseases!

His YouTube Channel and Twitter Account
https://www.youtube.com/@anthonychaffeemd

https://twitter.com/anthony_chaffee

Made in the USA
Monee, IL
03 November 2023

45738376R00075

Advance Praise for Divine Warrior Training

Divine Warrior Training is a wonderful book! I am honored that my music is often used in the circles Thomas facilitates for people to live into their potential.

    Peter Kater, Pianist-Composer
    www.peterkater.com

Thomas Capshew's book Divine Warrior Training is a foundational work for anyone who has found themselves on the path of self-discovery. The easy manner in which this book presents its information will almost seem simplistic at times, but that's the place to start. Reading Thomas' words about his history and his journey will provide insights into the difficulty of the journey and, more importantly, the bliss of the journey. The information is presented in a calm and reassuring manner to let the reader know that those that stay the course will have great rewards that can then be shared with the world. Thomas' questions at the back of the book are not frivolous. He challenges the reader to dig deep so that they may find their roots and grow to their fullest and, in doing so, bless us all.

    Patrick Hundt, La Crosse, Wisconsin

Divine Warrior Training is a brilliant book and I loved it a bunch! I especially loved the chapter on the Christians among us."

    David K. Banner, Ph.D.
    Author of *Frameshifting: A Path to Wholeness*

Advance Praise for Divine Warrior Training

Thomas Capshew's book, Divine Warrior Training: Manifesting the Divine in our World, is destined to be among the current handful of texts that are essential reads and studies for those of us who are involved in the conscious process of awakening to full awareness and self-evolution from human to divine. The transforming information this book imparts is easy both to comprehend and to activate, using the effective exercise tools provided. Thank you Thomas for answering your own divine calling to warriorship.

    Carlos W. Anderson, Minister, Teacher, Composer, Healer
    Author of *OPEN TO THE MAGIC! Beyond Religion and into the Mind of Christ*. www.onelifeschool.com

Elegant, direct, and loving, Divine Warrior Training transmits a powerful message with adamantine strength and crystal clarity. These pages contain an inspiring, fresh perspective on consciousness accompanied by a thoughtful collection of exercises to implement real personal transformation. Divine Warrior Training is an invitation to set aside fear and unleash the spiritual warrior within!!

    Kalleen Ragan-Pepper, LMSW
    Paths to Empowerment workshops

Advance Praise for Divine Warrior Training

I sat down and read Divine Warrior Training cover to cover in one sitting! The book is wonderful, simply wonderful. It puts into words all the things I've felt for years. Being a divine warrior allows you to sweep away all the cobwebs of religions and the hindrance of human limitation - it sets one free. I am so joyful right now - I DO remember who I am. I AM a divine warrior. Thank you.
    Corky Severson

As most of us know, we can read about and intellectually embrace a spiritual concept, but to actually "do the work" to incorporate that concept into our lives is another story. In Divine Warrior Training, Thomas Capshew provides clear guidance, helping us to actually do the work we need to do. In this easy to grasp yet profoundly empowering book, Capshew gently encourages us to explore our edges and move into those "shadow" areas of our lives that we would otherwise choose not to visit. We are reminded that, "the most powerful force that humans have is the power of choice... Choice can move us toward the divine and choice is what can keep us separated from the divine." Part reader, part resource guide, part workbook, Divine Warrior Training is a valuable asset to anyone exploring the realms of conscious spiritual growth.
    Andrea Garvey, Editor
    Creations Magazine, Northport, New York
    www.creationsmagazine.com

I love how simply the book reads. I appreciate how Thomas takes what could easily have been a very abstract, obscure and difficult array of concepts and distills them into incredibly lucid, easily ingestible language.
    Matt Coffman

Advance Praise for Divine Warrior Training

I have just finished reading the book and it was so wonderful. Many, many parts spoke directly to my soul and resonated so deeply within me.
    Nicole Hoag

We are all looking for how and where we fit into the world, and how we can live together on this planet. Thomas Capshew's new book Divine Warrior Training offers each of us concepts, ideas and skills to help us find that very special place that is our own and yet create a path towards light and love for all the peoples of this planet. Utilizing universal concepts and personal exercises, all of us can become Divine Warriors and bring peace to ourselves and the world in our lifetime.
    Rev. Deborah Ross and Rabbi Roger Ross, Directors
    The New Seminary for Interfaith Studies
    New York, New York

In a world so lacking vision, wisdom, kindness, love, joy, peace, and generosity, Thomas Capshew has written a book about coming into a relationship with the divine, no matter what path you have chosen to get there. Christian brothers and sisters willing to search for truth in new and progressive ways will find here a wonderful introduction into a more "…expansive awareness of Jesus' life and words." The book includes concrete steps - Divine Warrior Training Exercises - which can be taken by the reader to enhance the experience. I found it to be an easy read, yet profoundly challenging. I highly recommend it.
    Rev. Joel Love, Pastor
    Union Congregational United Church of Christ
    Reinbeck, Iowa